Chapter 1: Introduction to Aldosterone

The Role of Aldosterone in the Human Body

Aldosterone is a vital hormone that plays a critical role in regulating various bodily functions. As part of the steroid hormone family, aldosterone is produced in the adrenal glands, specifically in the zona glomerulosa of the adrenal cortex. It is primarily involved in the regulation of fluid and electrolyte balance, influencing the amount of sodium and potassium in the body. This regulation is crucial because it helps maintain blood pressure, fluid volume, and the body's overall homeostasis. Without proper aldosterone functioning, serious health issues can arise, such as imbalanced blood pressure, dehydration, or even organ damage.

Aldosterone's main action occurs in the kidneys, where it stimulates sodium retention and potassium excretion, a process that directly affects blood volume and pressure. It works by binding to mineralocorticoid receptors in the renal tubules, prompting the reabsorption of sodium from the urine back into the bloodstream. This action not only retains sodium but also indirectly retains water due to osmosis, which leads to an increase in blood volume. Meanwhile, potassium, which must be kept in check for proper cellular function, is excreted into the urine.

Though aldosterone's effects are most commonly associated with the kidneys, its influence extends throughout the body. It affects the cardiovascular system, the brain, and even plays a role in stress responses. Aldosterone's actions can be influenced by various factors, such as blood pressure, sodium intake, and hormonal signals, and its levels fluctuate throughout the day to meet the body's ever-changing needs.

Aldosterone's Importance in Hormonal Balance

The human body is a finely tuned machine, and aldosterone plays a central role in maintaining the delicate hormonal balance required for optimal functioning. As part of the broader endocrine system, aldosterone works in concert with other hormones to regulate key functions such as metabolism, immune response, and stress adaptation. While aldosterone is best known for its impact on fluid balance and blood pressure, its interactions with other hormones such as cortisol, insulin, and parathyroid hormone highlight its broader influence.

The aldosterone-cortisol connection, in particular, is significant because both hormones are produced in the adrenal glands and share a common precursor, cholesterol. Cortisol is known for its role in the body's stress response, regulating metabolism and the immune system. When the body encounters stress, cortisol and aldosterone levels often rise together. Cortisol increases blood sugar and suppresses inflammation, while aldosterone ensures the body retains sufficient sodium and water, supporting cardiovascular health during times of physical or emotional strain.

Aldosterone's role in electrolyte balance further underscores its importance in hormonal health. Its ability to regulate sodium and potassium ensures the proper functioning of every cell in the body, from nerve conduction to muscle contraction. Even slight imbalances in these electrolytes can lead to severe consequences, including arrhythmias, muscle weakness, and neurological disturbances.

In this way, aldosterone is not just a hormone for fluid regulation, but a key player in maintaining the equilibrium of multiple systems that are essential for life. Its impact on other hormones makes it central to understanding the broader picture of health, particularly with conditions such as hypertension, heart failure, and kidney disease, where aldosterone dysregulation is often at play.

Understanding the Renin-Angiotensin-Aldosterone System (RAAS)

The renin-angiotensin-aldosterone system (RAAS) is the body's key regulatory mechanism for blood pressure and fluid balance. The system's role is to detect changes in blood pressure and volume and respond by releasing aldosterone to correct any imbalances. The RAAS system is activated when the kidneys sense a drop in blood pressure or sodium levels. In response, they release an enzyme called renin into the bloodstream.

Renin then acts on a protein called angiotensinogen, which is produced by the liver and circulates in the blood. Renin converts angiotensinogen into angiotensin I, which is subsequently converted into angiotensin II by the enzyme angiotensin-converting enzyme (ACE), primarily in the lungs. Angiotensin II has several critical effects on the body: it constricts blood vessels, raising blood pressure, and it stimulates the adrenal glands to release aldosterone.

Aldosterone, in turn, acts on the kidneys to retain sodium and water, increasing blood volume and, subsequently, blood pressure. This cascade of events illustrates how tightly blood pressure and fluid balance are regulated through hormonal signals. RAAS plays a fundamental role in responding to low blood pressure, dehydration, or sodium imbalance, making aldosterone a vital player in maintaining normal physiological conditions.

Interestingly, in conditions such as primary hyperaldosteronism (Conn's syndrome), where there is overproduction of aldosterone, this system becomes overactive. The excessive retention of sodium and water can lead to elevated blood pressure (hypertension), which is one of the hallmark symptoms of the disorder. Understanding the RAAS system is crucial not only for understanding aldosterone's normal function but also for recognizing when it is dysregulated, as in various cardiovascular and renal diseases.

In conclusion, aldosterone is much more than just a regulator of salt and water balance; it is a key player in maintaining the overall stability of the body's internal environment. Its effects on the kidneys, cardiovascular system, and electrolyte balance make it indispensable for health. In the chapters that follow, we will delve deeper into the physiological mechanisms that govern aldosterone's actions, its impact on various organ systems, and how its regulation can be influenced by factors ranging from diet and exercise to disease and aging. By understanding aldosterone, we unlock the ability to manage our health more effectively and ensure the proper functioning of this crucial hormone system.

Chapter 2: The Physiological Mechanisms of Aldosterone
How Aldosterone Affects the Kidneys and Sodium Reabsorption

Aldosterone plays an essential role in maintaining fluid and electrolyte balance in the body, and one of its primary targets is the kidneys. The kidneys are responsible for filtering the blood, removing waste products, and regulating important substances like sodium, potassium, and water. Aldosterone's action on the kidneys is vital for regulating blood pressure and maintaining homeostasis.

Aldosterone exerts its effects by binding to mineralocorticoid receptors located in the distal tubules and collecting ducts of the kidneys. This binding triggers a series of events that lead to the reabsorption of sodium from the urine back into the bloodstream. As sodium is reabsorbed, water naturally follows due to osmotic forces, which increases blood volume. This rise in blood volume, in turn, helps to raise blood pressure.

In addition to sodium, aldosterone also affects the movement of other electrolytes, particularly potassium. The reabsorption of sodium in exchange for potassium occurs in the renal tubules, making aldosterone a key player in both sodium retention and potassium excretion. This process ensures that the body retains sufficient sodium while maintaining appropriate potassium levels, which are critical for cellular function, nerve transmission, and muscle contraction.

Without aldosterone's regulatory actions, the kidneys would not be able to balance the levels of sodium and water, leading to disturbances in blood pressure, fluid balance, and overall electrolyte homeostasis. This explains why aldosterone is so closely associated with the regulation of blood pressure.

Aldosterone and Potassium Regulation

In addition to its well-known role in sodium retention, aldosterone is also crucial in regulating potassium levels in the body. Potassium is a key electrolyte involved in the proper function of cells, nerves, and muscles, particularly in maintaining cellular resting potentials and ensuring proper electrical activity in the heart. Too much potassium in the blood (hyperkalemia) or too little potassium (hypokalemia) can result in serious health complications, including arrhythmias, muscle weakness, and even paralysis.

Aldosterone's influence on potassium regulation occurs in the same renal cells where it promotes sodium retention. Specifically, aldosterone stimulates the sodium-potassium ATPase pump in the distal nephron cells, increasing the exchange of sodium for potassium. This results in the excretion of excess potassium in the urine. As a result, aldosterone plays a vital role in maintaining potassium homeostasis by ensuring that any excess potassium is removed from the body, thus preventing harmful accumulation.

The balance between sodium and potassium is carefully maintained to support normal cellular function, and aldosterone is central to this regulation. For example, in states of aldosterone deficiency, potassium levels can rise, leading to hyperkalemia, which is often seen in conditions like Addison's disease. Conversely, in cases of excessive aldosterone production, such as in primary hyperaldosteronism, potassium levels can drop, leading to hypokalemia, which is characterized by muscle weakness, cramps, and fatigue.

The Aldosterone and Blood Pressure Connection

One of the most significant roles of aldosterone is its effect on blood pressure regulation. The hormone is a key player in the body's response to blood volume and pressure changes. Aldosterone works in conjunction with the renin-angiotensin-aldosterone system (RAAS), a feedback system that helps maintain blood pressure and fluid balance. The activation of RAAS in response to low blood pressure or sodium levels leads to the release of aldosterone from the adrenal glands.

Once released, aldosterone stimulates the kidneys to retain sodium and water, which increases the volume of blood circulating through the body. This rise in blood volume subsequently raises blood pressure, helping to restore normal levels. In this way, aldosterone acts as a regulator of long-term blood pressure by influencing sodium and water retention.

Aldosterone's impact on blood pressure is particularly important in situations of dehydration or blood loss. For example, when the body experiences a drop in blood pressure, such as during a hemorrhage or dehydration, aldosterone helps to increase blood volume and prevent a dangerous drop in blood pressure. Similarly, aldosterone's role in maintaining blood pressure extends to its regulation of sodium intake, as the hormone ensures that the body holds on to sodium during times of fluid deficit, thus preventing further drops in blood pressure.

Excess aldosterone production, however, can lead to high blood pressure, a condition known as hyperaldosteronism or Conn's syndrome. In this disorder, the excessive reabsorption of sodium and water results in an increase in blood volume and hypertension. The elevated blood pressure, in turn, places additional strain on the cardiovascular system and increases the risk of heart disease, stroke, and kidney damage.

Conversely, aldosterone deficiency can contribute to low blood pressure (hypotension). This occurs when the kidneys fail to retain adequate sodium and water, resulting in decreased blood volume and lower pressure. Conditions like Addison's disease, where aldosterone levels are deficient, can cause hypotension, dizziness, and fainting, as the body is unable to effectively regulate blood pressure.

Thus, aldosterone's effect on blood pressure is a balancing act that requires precise regulation. Both high and low levels of aldosterone can lead to cardiovascular complications, which makes understanding and managing aldosterone levels crucial in maintaining cardiovascular health.

Conclusion

Aldosterone is a powerful hormone that plays an indispensable role in regulating fluid balance, electrolyte homeostasis, and blood pressure. By acting on the kidneys, it promotes sodium retention, potassium excretion, and water reabsorption, which helps maintain blood volume and pressure. Through its interactions with the RAAS system, aldosterone ensures that the body responds appropriately to changes in blood pressure, such as during dehydration or blood loss. However, when aldosterone is dysregulated— whether through overproduction or deficiency—it can contribute to a range of serious health issues, including hypertension, electrolyte imbalances, and cardiovascular complications.

Understanding how aldosterone functions in the body is essential for mastering its role in health and disease. In the following chapters, we will explore how aldosterone's production is regulated, its effects on various organ systems, and the disorders that arise when aldosterone levels are too high or too low. By gaining a deeper understanding of aldosterone's physiological mechanisms, we can better manage our health and address the conditions associated with aldosterone dysregulation.

Chapter 3: Aldosterone Secretion and Regulation
How Aldosterone Is Produced and Released

Aldosterone is synthesized and secreted by the adrenal glands, which are located on top of the kidneys. Specifically, aldosterone is produced in the zona glomerulosa, the outermost layer of the adrenal cortex. The production of aldosterone is tightly regulated by a variety of physiological mechanisms to ensure that it responds appropriately to the body's needs, particularly in maintaining fluid balance, blood pressure, and electrolyte homeostasis.

The synthesis of aldosterone begins with cholesterol, which is converted into pregnenolone, the precursor for all steroid hormones. Pregnenolone is then converted into mineralocorticoid hormones, including aldosterone. The process is influenced by several factors, most notably the activation of the renin-angiotensin-aldosterone system (RAAS), which plays a central role in regulating aldosterone production.

Aldosterone is released into the bloodstream in response to several stimuli, such as low blood pressure, low sodium levels, or high potassium levels. Once released, it travels through the blood and binds to mineralocorticoid receptors in target tissues, primarily the kidneys, where it exerts its effects. Aldosterone's action on the kidneys involves promoting sodium retention and potassium excretion, both of which contribute to blood pressure regulation and fluid balance.

Factors That Trigger Aldosterone Release

Aldosterone secretion is primarily regulated by the renin-angiotensin-aldosterone system (RAAS), but several other factors can also influence its release. These include changes in blood volume, electrolyte concentrations, and hormonal signals.

1. **Renin-Angiotensin-Aldosterone System (RAAS):**

   The RAAS is the most powerful regulator of aldosterone secretion. When blood pressure or sodium levels drop, or when potassium levels rise, the kidneys sense these changes and release the enzyme renin. Renin acts on angiotensinogen, a protein produced by the liver, converting it into angiotensin I. Angiotensin I is then converted to angiotensin II by the enzyme angiotensin-converting enzyme (ACE), primarily in the lungs. Angiotensin II stimulates aldosterone release from the adrenal glands. Additionally, angiotensin II directly causes vasoconstriction, raising blood pressure.

2. **Potassium Levels:**

   Elevated potassium levels in the blood (hyperkalemia) are a potent trigger for aldosterone release. Aldosterone acts to excrete excess potassium through the kidneys, restoring normal potassium balance. Conversely, low potassium levels (hypokalemia) suppress aldosterone secretion.

3. **Sodium Levels:**

   Low sodium levels (hyponatremia) also stimulate aldosterone release through the RAAS. In this case, aldosterone promotes the reabsorption of sodium in the kidneys, thereby increasing sodium levels in the blood. Conversely, high sodium levels (hypernatremia) typically reduce aldosterone release, as the body seeks to prevent further sodium retention.

4. **Blood Volume and Blood Pressure:**

   When the body experiences low blood volume, as in the case of dehydration or blood loss, aldosterone is released to help restore blood volume by promoting sodium and water retention. In conditions of high blood pressure, aldosterone secretion may be suppressed to prevent excessive fluid retention and further elevation of blood pressure.

5. **Adrenocorticotropic Hormone (ACTH):**

   Although its effect is less significant than the RAAS, ACTH, a hormone produced by the pituitary gland, can also stimulate aldosterone release. ACTH is primarily involved in cortisol secretion but has a mild effect on aldosterone production, particularly during periods of stress.

Feedback Mechanisms in Aldosterone Secretion

Aldosterone secretion is tightly controlled by feedback mechanisms that maintain homeostasis within the body. These feedback loops ensure that aldosterone levels rise when needed to restore balance, and fall when the body has achieved sufficient sodium and water retention. Several important feedback systems regulate aldosterone release:

1. **RAAS Feedback Loop:**

   The RAAS system itself operates through a negative feedback mechanism. When aldosterone is released in response to a drop in blood pressure or sodium levels, its effects lead to increased sodium and water retention, which raises blood volume and pressure. Once normal blood pressure or sodium levels are restored, the stimulus for renin release decreases, reducing aldosterone production and creating a self-regulating loop.

2. **Potassium Feedback:**

   Potassium plays a key role in aldosterone regulation. When blood potassium levels are high, aldosterone is released to promote potassium excretion by the kidneys. As potassium levels normalize, aldosterone secretion decreases, completing the feedback loop.

3. **Natriuretic Peptides:**

   When blood pressure or blood volume rises, the heart releases hormones called natriuretic peptides (e.g., atrial natriuretic peptide or BNP). These hormones inhibit aldosterone release by opposing the effects of RAAS. They promote sodium excretion and vasodilation, counteracting the effects of aldosterone and reducing blood volume and pressure.

4. **Adrenal Feedback Mechanism:**

   The adrenal glands themselves also respond to aldosterone levels. High aldosterone levels can inhibit the further secretion of aldosterone through a negative feedback mechanism within the adrenal cortex. This helps prevent the overproduction of aldosterone, ensuring that levels remain within an optimal range.

Aldosterone in Fluid Balance

Aldosterone's most prominent role is in fluid balance, which is essential for maintaining normal blood pressure and cellular function. By regulating sodium and water retention in the kidneys, aldosterone helps to maintain blood volume and pressure, ensuring that tissues receive adequate hydration and that waste products are efficiently excreted.

When the body experiences dehydration or low blood pressure, aldosterone is released to promote sodium retention in the kidneys. As sodium is reabsorbed, water follows, leading to an increase in blood volume and pressure. This is particularly important during periods of stress, illness, or blood loss when maintaining adequate blood flow to organs and tissues is critical.

However, when fluid levels are sufficient, aldosterone release is suppressed to prevent excessive sodium and water retention, which could lead to fluid overload and elevated blood pressure. This delicate balance is crucial for maintaining optimal health.

In addition to regulating fluid balance, aldosterone also influences other systems in the body. For example, its effects on the cardiovascular system include helping to maintain normal heart function by balancing fluid levels and supporting blood pressure regulation. In the brain, aldosterone influences the hypothalamus and pituitary gland, helping to coordinate stress responses and the release of other hormones.

Conclusion

Aldosterone's production and secretion are carefully regulated by a variety of mechanisms that ensure the body maintains optimal fluid balance, blood pressure, and electrolyte homeostasis. The renin-angiotensin-aldosterone system (RAAS) plays the most significant role in stimulating aldosterone release in response to changes in blood volume, sodium levels, and potassium levels. Additionally, aldosterone release is subject to feedback regulation by potassium, sodium, and natriuretic peptides, helping to maintain equilibrium.

Understanding how aldosterone is produced and regulated is critical for managing conditions related to blood pressure, fluid balance, and electrolyte imbalances. In the next chapters, we will explore how aldosterone's actions influence various body systems and how dysregulation of aldosterone can lead to disorders such as hypertension, kidney disease, and heart failure. By mastering aldosterone's secretion and regulation, we can better understand its role in maintaining health and preventing disease.

Chapter 4: Aldosterone in Fluid Balance
How Aldosterone Controls Sodium and Water Retention

One of aldosterone's most critical roles in the body is its regulation of sodium and water balance. By influencing the kidneys, aldosterone ensures that the body maintains an adequate volume of blood and tissues remain hydrated, both of which are essential for normal cellular function, organ performance, and overall homeostasis.

When aldosterone is released from the adrenal glands, it acts on the distal tubules and collecting ducts of the kidneys. In these areas, it binds to specific mineralocorticoid receptors, initiating a process that promotes the reabsorption of sodium from the urine back into the bloodstream. Sodium, in turn, attracts water due to osmosis, causing water to follow sodium back into the bloodstream. This retention of sodium and water helps increase blood volume, thereby contributing to the maintenance of blood pressure.

Aldosterone's influence on sodium reabsorption is particularly important in the context of dehydration or low blood volume. When the body detects a drop in blood pressure or dehydration, aldosterone is released to preserve sodium and water, restoring fluid balance and ensuring that organs receive adequate circulation. In this way, aldosterone plays a crucial role in preventing hypovolemia (low blood volume), which can lead to dizziness, fainting, and organ failure if not properly managed.

This sodium and water retention mechanism also helps prevent electrolyte imbalances. Since sodium is a key regulator of extracellular fluid volume, aldosterone's ability to maintain sodium levels is critical for avoiding both dehydration and fluid overload.

The Role of Aldosterone in Dehydration and Overhydration

Aldosterone's impact on fluid balance becomes particularly apparent during periods of dehydration or overhydration.

1. **Dehydration**:

   When the body experiences dehydration, often due to excessive fluid loss (e.g., sweating, vomiting, diarrhea), blood volume decreases, which triggers a cascade of hormonal signals to restore balance. Aldosterone, through its action on the kidneys, ensures that sodium—and, by extension, water—are reabsorbed into the bloodstream, helping to restore blood volume and prevent further fluid loss. This compensatory response is crucial for survival, particularly in conditions where fluid loss is rapid or severe.

   Additionally, dehydration can activate the RAAS system, further boosting aldosterone secretion and intensifying the retention of sodium and water. This response can help restore the balance between blood volume and electrolyte concentrations, preventing hypotension (low blood pressure) and supporting proper organ function.

2. Overhydration:

On the other hand, when there is excess fluid in the body (often due to excessive intake of water or fluid retention associated with certain medical conditions), aldosterone works to prevent overhydration by reducing sodium retention. With less sodium reabsorbed by the kidneys, water follows and is excreted, helping to decrease blood volume and restore normal fluid levels. In situations of overhydration, aldosterone levels may be suppressed to avoid excessive fluid retention that could lead to edema (fluid accumulation in tissues) or hypertension.

Aldosterone's regulation of fluid balance is not just about responding to changes in water intake but also about responding to the body's need for sodium and the effects that sodium levels have on water retention. By finely tuning sodium reabsorption, aldosterone ensures that the body does not lose too much water during dehydration or hold on to too much water in the case of fluid overload.

Impact of Aldosterone on Blood Volume

Blood volume is a critical determinant of blood pressure, and aldosterone plays a key role in ensuring that blood volume remains within a range that supports proper circulation and tissue perfusion. When aldosterone levels are high, more sodium and water are reabsorbed by the kidneys, leading to increased blood volume. This is especially important when blood volume is low, such as in the case of blood loss, dehydration, or certain cardiovascular conditions.

By increasing blood volume, aldosterone directly helps to stabilize blood pressure. For instance, in the case of a sudden drop in blood pressure due to hemorrhage or dehydration, aldosterone's action to increase blood volume can be a life-saving response. However, when aldosterone production is excessive or dysregulated, it can lead to increased blood volume and elevated blood pressure, contributing to conditions such as hypertension, heart disease, and kidney dysfunction.

This is why aldosterone is sometimes referred to as a "blood volume regulator"—it maintains an optimal volume of circulating blood to ensure that tissues receive adequate oxygen and nutrients while also preventing damage to blood vessels that could occur with excessively high or low blood volume.

Aldosterone and Blood Pressure Control

The relationship between aldosterone and blood pressure is one of the most well-studied aspects of its function. Aldosterone's ability to influence sodium and water retention in the kidneys means that it has a direct effect on blood pressure. When blood pressure is low or when the body perceives a drop in blood volume, aldosterone is released to promote sodium and water retention, which raises blood volume and blood pressure.

Conversely, when blood pressure is too high, aldosterone secretion is often suppressed as part of a feedback loop that reduces sodium retention and encourages sodium excretion. In this way, aldosterone works in tandem with other mechanisms—such as the renin-angiotensin-aldosterone system (RAAS), the natriuretic peptides, and the autonomic nervous system—to fine-tune blood pressure regulation.

This fine-tuning becomes critically important in the context of hypertension. In individuals with primary hyperaldosteronism (Conn's syndrome), an overproduction of aldosterone leads to excessive sodium retention, which increases blood volume and raises blood pressure. Conversely, in individuals with aldosterone deficiency, the body may struggle to retain sufficient sodium and water, potentially leading to low blood pressure and symptoms of dehydration.

By controlling blood volume and pressure through its actions on the kidneys, aldosterone plays an essential role in the body's ability to maintain an optimal internal environment, ensuring that organs and tissues receive adequate blood flow under varying physiological conditions.

Conclusion

Aldosterone is a key player in fluid balance, directly influencing the retention of sodium and water in the kidneys. Its regulation of blood volume helps stabilize blood pressure, preventing both hypotension and hypertension. By responding to changes in hydration status, blood volume, and electrolyte levels, aldosterone ensures that the body maintains optimal fluid balance and blood pressure.

In the next chapters, we will explore how aldosterone dysregulation, whether through overproduction or deficiency, can contribute to a range of health conditions, including hypertension, kidney disease, and heart failure. Additionally, we will discuss the clinical management of aldosterone-related disorders, exploring both pharmacological and lifestyle interventions that can help maintain a healthy balance. By understanding aldosterone's role in fluid and blood pressure regulation, we gain valuable insight into the body's broader mechanisms for maintaining homeostasis and preventing disease.

Chapter 5: Aldosterone and Blood Pressure Control

The Link Between Aldosterone and Hypertension

Aldosterone is intricately connected to blood pressure regulation, and its role in hypertension (high blood pressure) has been well-established in both physiological and clinical settings. As a hormone responsible for regulating sodium and water balance in the kidneys, aldosterone directly influences blood volume—one of the key determinants of blood pressure. When aldosterone levels are elevated, sodium and water are retained, which increases blood volume and, consequently, raises blood pressure.

Hypertension, especially when linked to aldosterone overproduction, presents significant risks to cardiovascular health. Long-standing high blood pressure can cause damage to blood vessels, leading to an increased risk of stroke, heart attack, kidney failure, and other severe complications. Understanding the link between aldosterone and hypertension is crucial for both the prevention and treatment of these conditions.

The most common form of aldosterone-driven hypertension is primary hyperaldosteronism (also known as Conn's syndrome), where the adrenal glands produce excessive amounts of aldosterone, leading to high blood pressure. In these cases, the increase in blood pressure is largely due to the retention of sodium and water, which boosts blood volume and pressure, while simultaneously causing potassium depletion, which can result in various clinical manifestations.

How Aldosterone Increases Blood Pressure

Aldosterone's effect on blood pressure begins with its influence on the kidneys. By promoting sodium retention and water reabsorption, aldosterone increases blood volume, which directly raises blood pressure. The mechanism behind this involves the activation of sodium channels and sodium-potassium ATPase pumps in the kidneys, which allow sodium to be reabsorbed back into the bloodstream.

The retention of sodium in the kidneys also triggers a series of other events that contribute to increased blood pressure:

1. **Water Retention:**

   Sodium is a key factor in regulating fluid balance. When sodium is retained in the kidneys, water follows due to osmotic forces, increasing blood volume and pressure.

2. **Increased Blood Volume:**

   As the kidneys retain more sodium and water, the total volume of blood circulating through the body rises. This increased volume leads to higher pressure against the walls of the blood vessels, a key factor in the development of hypertension.

3. **Vasoconstriction:**

   Aldosterone also indirectly increases blood pressure through vasoconstriction, the narrowing of blood vessels. Although this effect is primarily driven by the angiotensin II component of the RAAS (renin-angiotensin-aldosterone system), aldosterone can further contribute to increased vascular resistance, making it harder for blood to flow through the vessels and further elevating blood pressure.

4. **Potassium Loss:**

   High aldosterone levels also increase potassium excretion through the kidneys. The imbalance between sodium and potassium can affect the electrical function of the heart and blood vessels, contributing to arrhythmias and exacerbating hypertension.

Overall, aldosterone acts as a key player in maintaining blood pressure by regulating sodium and fluid balance. However, when its secretion becomes dysregulated, as in primary hyperaldosteronism, it can lead to pathologically high blood pressure that is difficult to control without medical intervention.

Addressing the Effects of High Aldosterone

Managing high aldosterone levels involves targeting both the hormone itself and the mechanisms by which it influences blood pressure. There are several approaches to address the effects of elevated aldosterone, ranging from pharmacological interventions to lifestyle modifications.

1. **Aldosterone Antagonists (Mineralocorticoid Receptor Antagonists):**

   One of the primary treatments for high aldosterone levels and the associated hypertension is the use of aldosterone antagonists, such as **spironolactone** and **eplerenone**. These drugs block the mineralocorticoid receptors in the kidneys, preventing aldosterone from binding and exerting its effects. As a result, sodium retention is reduced, and potassium levels are more effectively maintained. Spironolactone, in particular, is widely used not only for treating hypertension but also for heart failure, as it has been shown to reduce the risk of cardiovascular events.

2. **Angiotensin-Converting Enzyme (ACE) Inhibitors and Angiotensin II Receptor Blockers (ARBs):**

   These classes of drugs work by inhibiting the action of angiotensin II, the hormone that stimulates aldosterone release. By reducing angiotensin II activity, ACE inhibitors and ARBs can decrease aldosterone secretion, lower blood pressure, and reduce the effects of excessive aldosterone. These drugs are often used in conjunction with aldosterone antagonists in patients with resistant hypertension or heart failure.

3. **Dietary Modifications:**

   Reducing sodium intake is one of the most straightforward ways to mitigate the effects of high aldosterone levels. Since aldosterone's main action is to retain sodium, cutting back on dietary sodium helps reduce the amount of sodium that needs to be retained by the kidneys. This can be beneficial for managing blood pressure, particularly in individuals who are salt-sensitive or have hyperaldosteronism. Additionally, increasing potassium intake through dietary sources (such as bananas, oranges, and leafy greens) can help counteract the potassium loss induced by aldosterone.

4. **Lifestyle Changes:**

   In addition to dietary modifications, lifestyle factors such as weight loss, regular exercise, and stress reduction can also help lower blood pressure and improve overall cardiovascular health. For individuals with hypertension related to high aldosterone levels, adopting a healthy lifestyle is an essential part of the treatment plan.

5. **Surgical Intervention (in cases of adenomas):**

In some cases of primary hyperaldosteronism, the underlying cause is an aldosterone-producing adenoma (a benign tumor of the adrenal gland). If the tumor is localized and accessible, surgical removal may be necessary to treat the condition and restore normal aldosterone levels. In cases where the adenoma cannot be surgically removed, medical management with aldosterone antagonists and other antihypertensive medications is typically employed.

Managing Primary Hyperaldosteronism (Conn's Syndrome)

Primary hyperaldosteronism, also known as Conn's syndrome, is a condition characterized by the excessive production of aldosterone, usually due to an adrenal adenoma or bilateral adrenal hyperplasia. It leads to chronic hypertension, hypokalemia (low potassium), and metabolic alkalosis (increased blood pH). Symptoms may include muscle weakness, fatigue, headaches, and excessive thirst.

1. **Diagnosis:**

   The diagnosis of primary hyperaldosteronism involves measuring plasma aldosterone and renin levels. An aldosterone-to-renin ratio (ARR) is often used as an initial screening tool. If the ratio is elevated, further testing such as confirmatory saline infusion tests or adrenal imaging may be performed to identify the source of excess aldosterone production.

2. **Treatment:**

   For those with adrenal adenomas, surgical removal is often the treatment of choice. In cases of bilateral adrenal hyperplasia, where both adrenal glands are overproducing aldosterone, medical therapy with aldosterone antagonists is the mainstay of treatment. Lifestyle changes, including reducing sodium intake and managing stress, are also recommended to help control blood pressure.

Conclusion

Aldosterone plays a critical role in regulating blood pressure by modulating sodium and water balance. When aldosterone production is dysregulated, it can lead to conditions such as primary hyperaldosteronism and hypertension. Managing elevated aldosterone levels involves a combination of pharmacological treatments, dietary changes, and lifestyle modifications. By addressing the underlying causes of high aldosterone and using appropriate therapies, it is possible to control blood pressure and reduce the risk of cardiovascular complications. In the following chapters, we will explore the impact of aldosterone on other organ systems, including the kidneys, heart, and brain, and discuss advanced strategies for managing aldosterone-related disorders.

Chapter 6: Disorders of Aldosterone Production

Aldosterone is a key regulator of fluid balance, sodium and potassium levels, and blood pressure. However, when the body produces too much or too little aldosterone, it can lead to a range of disorders that impact health. Understanding the underlying causes and treatment options for these disorders is crucial for maintaining optimal health. In this chapter, we will explore two major disorders related to aldosterone production: primary aldosteronism (Conn's syndrome) and secondary hyperaldosteronism. We will also discuss the consequences of aldosterone deficiency and the impact of low aldosterone on electrolyte balance.

Primary Aldosteronism (Conn's Syndrome)

Primary aldosteronism, also known as Conn's syndrome, is a condition characterized by the overproduction of aldosterone by the adrenal glands. This condition is typically caused by either an aldosterone-producing adenoma (a benign tumor of the adrenal gland) or, in some cases, bilateral adrenal hyperplasia (enlargement of both adrenal glands). The excessive aldosterone secretion leads to sodium and water retention, which increases blood volume and raises blood pressure.

Symptoms of Primary Aldosteronism:

- **Hypertension (high blood pressure):** Elevated aldosterone causes water and sodium retention, leading to an increase in blood volume and pressure.
- **Hypokalemia (low potassium levels):** Increased sodium reabsorption in the kidneys causes potassium to be excreted in excess, leading to low potassium levels.
- **Muscle weakness and cramps:** Low potassium levels can result in muscle weakness, fatigue, and cramps.
- **Frequent urination and excessive thirst:** Increased blood volume can lead to symptoms of dehydration and the need for frequent urination.
- **Headaches:** High blood pressure and electrolyte imbalances can contribute to headaches.

Diagnosis:

To diagnose primary aldosteronism, doctors typically measure the aldosterone-to-renin ratio (ARR) in the blood. An elevated ARR is a strong indicator of excessive aldosterone production. Further tests, including saline infusion tests and adrenal imaging, are often performed to confirm the diagnosis and identify the underlying cause, such as an adrenal adenoma or bilateral adrenal hyperplasia.

Treatment Options:

1. **Surgical Intervention (Adrenalectomy):**

   If the cause of primary aldosteronism is a unilateral aldosterone-producing adenoma, the treatment of choice is often surgical removal of the affected adrenal gland. This procedure is highly effective in normalizing blood pressure and restoring potassium balance.

2. **Medical Management (Aldosterone Antagonists):**

   For individuals with bilateral adrenal hyperplasia or those who cannot undergo surgery, medical treatment with aldosterone antagonists such as **spironolactone** or **eplerenone** is used. These medications block the effects of aldosterone by preventing it from binding to its receptors in the kidneys. This treatment helps reduce sodium retention, increase potassium levels, and manage blood pressure.

3. **Lifestyle Modifications:**

   Along with pharmacological treatment, dietary changes (such as reducing sodium intake and increasing potassium-rich foods) and lifestyle modifications (including regular exercise and stress management) are recommended to support blood pressure management.

Secondary Hyperaldosteronism

Secondary hyperaldosteronism is a condition in which aldosterone production is increased due to an underlying factor that stimulates the renin-angiotensin-aldosterone system (RAAS). Unlike primary aldosteronism, secondary hyperaldosteronism is not caused by a problem with the adrenal glands themselves but rather by external factors that trigger increased aldosterone secretion. Common causes of secondary hyperaldosteronism include:

- **Renal artery stenosis:** Narrowing of the renal arteries can lead to decreased blood flow to the kidneys, which activates RAAS and increases aldosterone production.
- **Congestive heart failure:** When the heart is unable to pump blood efficiently, blood flow to the kidneys is reduced, prompting RAAS activation and aldosterone release.
- **Cirrhosis of the liver:** Liver disease can cause fluid retention and reduce blood flow to the kidneys, leading to secondary hyperaldosteronism.
- **Nephrotic syndrome:** A kidney disorder that causes significant protein loss in the urine can activate RAAS and increase aldosterone secretion.
- **Pregnancy:** Increased blood volume during pregnancy can stimulate RAAS and cause elevated aldosterone levels, although this is a normal physiological response rather than a pathological one.

Symptoms of Secondary Hyperaldosteronism:

The symptoms of secondary hyperaldosteronism are similar to those of primary aldosteronism, as they both involve excessive aldosterone and its effects on sodium and water retention, blood pressure, and potassium excretion:

- Hypertension
- Hypokalemia
- Muscle weakness and cramps
- Increased thirst and urination
- Fatigue

Diagnosis:

Diagnosing secondary hyperaldosteronism typically involves measuring aldosterone and renin levels in the blood. A high aldosterone-to-renin ratio suggests secondary hyperaldosteronism, but further diagnostic testing is needed to determine the underlying cause. Imaging studies, such as ultrasound or CT scans, may be used to assess for conditions like renal artery stenosis or liver disease.

Treatment Options:

Treatment of secondary hyperaldosteronism focuses on addressing the underlying cause of the condition:

1. **Management of the Underlying Cause:**

   For conditions such as renal artery stenosis or heart failure, treating the primary condition (e.g., through surgery, angioplasty, or heart failure medications) can help normalize aldosterone levels.

2. **Aldosterone Antagonists:**

   Similar to primary aldosteronism, aldosterone antagonists like spironolactone or eplerenone may be used to block the effects of excess aldosterone and improve electrolyte balance and blood pressure.

3. **Lifestyle and Dietary Modifications:**

   Reducing sodium intake and increasing potassium intake are important steps in managing secondary hyperaldosteronism. Addressing lifestyle factors, such as improving cardiovascular health and managing stress, can also support treatment efforts.

Aldosterone Deficiency and Its Impact

Aldosterone deficiency occurs when the adrenal glands do not produce enough aldosterone. This condition is often seen in disorders such as **Addison's disease**, a primary adrenal insufficiency where both aldosterone and cortisol production are impaired. Aldosterone deficiency can lead to several symptoms due to the lack of sodium and water retention, resulting in imbalanced fluid levels and electrolytes.

Symptoms of Aldosterone Deficiency:

- **Hypotension (low blood pressure):** Without aldosterone, the kidneys are unable to retain sodium and water, leading to low blood volume and blood pressure.

- **Hyponatremia (low sodium levels):** The kidneys' inability to reabsorb sodium can lead to dangerously low levels of sodium in the blood.

- **Hyperkalemia (high potassium levels):** Without aldosterone, potassium is not excreted properly, leading to a dangerous buildup of potassium in the blood.

- **Fatigue and weakness:** Electrolyte imbalances and low blood pressure can lead to muscle weakness, dizziness, and fatigue.

- **Dehydration:** Inadequate sodium and water retention can result in dehydration, leading to symptoms such as dry skin, dry mouth, and excessive thirst.

Diagnosis:

Aldosterone deficiency is diagnosed through blood tests that measure sodium, potassium, and renin levels. Elevated renin levels in the presence of low aldosterone are indicative of adrenal insufficiency. Additional tests, such as ACTH stimulation tests and imaging studies, may be performed to confirm the diagnosis and identify the underlying cause.

Treatment:

Treatment of aldosterone deficiency typically involves:

1. **Aldosterone Replacement Therapy:**

   The primary treatment for aldosterone deficiency is hormone replacement, usually in the form of oral fludrocortisone, a synthetic corticosteroid that mimics aldosterone's effects. This medication helps to restore sodium and water retention, correct electrolyte imbalances, and stabilize blood pressure.

2. **Sodium and Fluid Management:**

   Individuals with aldosterone deficiency may need to increase their dietary salt intake and drink more fluids to help maintain blood volume and prevent dehydration.

3. **Monitoring and Lifestyle Adjustments:**

   Regular monitoring of blood pressure, electrolytes, and kidney function is essential. Lifestyle modifications, including avoiding excessive physical exertion and managing stress, can help prevent symptoms from worsening.

Conclusion

Disorders of aldosterone production, whether due to overproduction (primary and secondary hyperaldosteronism) or underproduction (aldosterone deficiency), can have significant effects on fluid balance, blood pressure, and electrolyte levels. Timely diagnosis and appropriate treatment are essential for managing these conditions and preventing complications such as cardiovascular disease, kidney damage, and stroke. By understanding the mechanisms behind these disorders and their treatment options, we can better manage aldosterone-related conditions and optimize overall health.

Chapter 7: Aldosterone Deficiency and Its Impact

Aldosterone is a vital hormone that plays a crucial role in maintaining fluid balance, blood pressure, and electrolyte homeostasis. When aldosterone production is insufficient, it leads to a deficiency that disrupts these systems, causing a wide range of physiological consequences. In this chapter, we will explore the causes and effects of aldosterone deficiency, with a focus on **Addison's disease** and the various impacts low aldosterone levels can have on electrolyte balance, hydration, and overall health.

Addison's Disease and Its Relationship to Aldosterone

Addison's disease, or primary adrenal insufficiency, is one of the most well-known causes of aldosterone deficiency. This autoimmune condition occurs when the adrenal glands are damaged and cannot produce adequate amounts of cortisol, aldosterone, or both. The most common causes of Addison's disease include autoimmune destruction of the adrenal glands, infections (such as tuberculosis), and other less common conditions, such as genetic disorders.

In Addison's disease, the impaired adrenal glands are unable to produce sufficient aldosterone. This leads to imbalances in sodium, potassium, and water regulation, which are critical for maintaining normal blood pressure and overall homeostasis.

Symptoms of Aldosterone Deficiency in Addison's Disease:

- **Hyponatremia (low sodium levels):** Aldosterone deficiency impairs the kidneys' ability to reabsorb sodium, leading to decreased sodium levels in the blood. This causes symptoms such as fatigue, weakness, dizziness, and, in severe cases, shock.

- **Hyperkalemia (high potassium levels):** Without aldosterone's effect on potassium excretion, potassium levels rise in the blood. Elevated potassium can lead to dangerous cardiac arrhythmias, muscle weakness, and, if left untreated, can be life-threatening.

- **Hypotension (low blood pressure):** Due to the loss of sodium and water, blood volume decreases, leading to low blood pressure. This can cause dizziness, fainting, and in severe cases, circulatory shock.

- **Dehydration:** The kidneys' inability to conserve water leads to dehydration, which exacerbates symptoms such as dry mouth, dark-colored urine, and excessive thirst.

- **Fatigue and Weight Loss:** The body's inability to properly regulate fluids and electrolytes can lead to general malaise, fatigue, and weight loss, which are hallmark symptoms of Addison's disease.

Diagnosis:

Aldosterone deficiency in Addison's disease is diagnosed through a series of blood tests that reveal low sodium, high potassium, and elevated renin levels. These findings are consistent with a lack of aldosterone production. Additional diagnostic tests, such as the ACTH (adrenocorticotropic hormone) stimulation test, can be performed to assess the adrenal glands' ability to produce cortisol and aldosterone in response to stress.

Treatment:

The primary treatment for aldosterone deficiency in Addison's disease is hormone replacement therapy. This typically involves:

- **Fludrocortisone:** A synthetic corticosteroid that mimics aldosterone's action in the body. It helps retain sodium, excrete potassium, and maintain blood pressure.

- **Hydrocortisone:** A synthetic form of cortisol is often used to replace the cortisol deficiency in Addison's disease, which also supports aldosterone's action to some extent.

- **Sodium and Fluid Management:** Patients with Addison's disease may be advised to increase their dietary sodium intake and consume more fluids, especially in hot climates or during periods of physical exertion, to prevent dehydration and maintain blood volume.

- **Stress Management:** During times of stress, illness, or injury, individuals with Addison's disease may require higher doses of cortisol and fludrocortisone to cope with the increased demands on their body.

In addition to hormone replacement, monitoring electrolyte levels, blood pressure, and kidney function is critical for managing aldosterone deficiency in Addison's disease. Regular follow-ups with healthcare providers are essential to adjust medication doses and prevent complications.

Effects of Low Aldosterone on Electrolyte Balance

Aldosterone plays a key role in regulating sodium and potassium levels in the body. When aldosterone levels are low, as in Addison's disease or other forms of adrenal insufficiency, the body is unable to maintain normal electrolyte balance, leading to significant disturbances.

Sodium Imbalance:

- Sodium is critical for maintaining fluid balance, blood pressure, and nerve function. In the absence of sufficient aldosterone, the kidneys cannot retain sodium, leading to **hyponatremia** (low sodium levels). This results in fluid shifts between the intracellular and extracellular spaces, causing dehydration and a reduction in blood volume.
- Hyponatremia can also cause symptoms such as dizziness, confusion, muscle cramps, and in severe cases, seizures and coma.

Potassium Imbalance:

- Aldosterone plays a crucial role in regulating potassium excretion by the kidneys. When aldosterone is deficient, potassium accumulates in the blood, leading to **hyperkalemia** (elevated potassium levels).

- High potassium levels can be dangerous, especially when they exceed the normal range. Symptoms of hyperkalemia include muscle weakness, fatigue, palpitations, and, in extreme cases, life-threatening arrhythmias.

- Hyperkalemia can also affect nerve conduction and muscular function, contributing to the fatigue and muscle weakness seen in aldosterone deficiency.

Chloride and Bicarbonate Imbalance:

- Aldosterone also helps regulate chloride and bicarbonate levels, which are important for maintaining acid-base balance. Low aldosterone levels can cause **metabolic acidosis**, a condition where the blood becomes too acidic due to the impaired regulation of bicarbonate and other buffering systems.

- Symptoms of metabolic acidosis include rapid breathing, confusion, and fatigue, and if left untreated, it can lead to serious complications such as kidney failure and respiratory distress.

Managing Aldosterone Deficiency

1. **Hormone Replacement Therapy:** The cornerstone of managing aldosterone deficiency is hormone replacement, particularly the use of fludrocortisone. This medication acts as a synthetic replacement for aldosterone, helping the kidneys retain sodium, excrete potassium, and maintain proper blood pressure and volume. In some cases, additional doses may be required during times of stress, such as illness, surgery, or physical exertion.

2. **Electrolyte and Fluid Management:** To help balance electrolyte levels, individuals with aldosterone deficiency may need to adjust their diet to include more sodium, especially during hot weather or when they are physically active. Ensuring adequate hydration is also vital for preventing dehydration and maintaining blood pressure.

3. **Regular Monitoring and Follow-Up Care:** Ongoing monitoring of electrolyte levels (sodium, potassium), blood pressure, and overall kidney function is essential for managing aldosterone deficiency. Regular follow-up appointments with healthcare providers allow for adjustments to treatment and timely intervention in case of any complications.

Conclusion

Aldosterone deficiency, whether caused by Addison's disease or other factors, can have a significant impact on fluid balance, blood pressure, and electrolyte levels. The resulting disturbances in sodium, potassium, and water regulation can lead to a variety of symptoms, including low blood pressure, dehydration, muscle weakness, and electrolyte imbalances. Timely diagnosis and appropriate treatment with aldosterone replacement therapy, electrolyte management, and regular monitoring are essential for managing aldosterone deficiency and improving quality of life. By understanding the mechanisms and consequences of aldosterone deficiency, we can better support individuals who are affected by this condition and help them maintain optimal health.

Chapter 8: Aldosterone Antagonists: Pharmacological Approaches

Aldosterone plays a pivotal role in regulating blood pressure, fluid balance, and electrolyte levels. However, when aldosterone is overproduced or becomes dysregulated, it can contribute to a range of disorders, including hypertension, heart failure, and kidney disease. To address these issues, aldosterone antagonists— medications that block the action of aldosterone—have been developed. In this chapter, we will explore the mechanisms of aldosterone antagonists, their use in clinical practice, their effectiveness in treating various conditions, and the side effects and considerations for their use.

Spironolactone and Eplerenone: Mechanisms of Action

Aldosterone antagonists work by blocking the mineralocorticoid receptors (MR) in the kidneys, heart, blood vessels, and brain, which are normally activated by aldosterone. By inhibiting this interaction, aldosterone antagonists prevent sodium retention, potassium excretion, and water reabsorption, which in turn helps reduce blood volume and blood pressure. The two most commonly used aldosterone antagonists are **spironolactone** and **eplerenone**.

Spironolactone:

Mechanism of Action:

Eplerenone:

Mechanism of Action:

Uses in Hypertension, Heart Failure, and Kidney Disease

Aldosterone antagonists have proven to be highly effective in managing several conditions associated with excessive aldosterone or fluid retention, including **hypertension, heart failure**, and **chronic kidney disease (CKD)**. Below are the key uses and benefits of these medications:

Hypertension (High Blood Pressure):

- **Role in Treatment:**

  Aldosterone antagonists help lower blood pressure by reducing sodium and water retention, thus decreasing blood volume and the overall workload on the heart. They are particularly beneficial in **resistant hypertension**, a condition where blood pressure remains elevated despite the use of multiple antihypertensive agents.

- **Effectiveness:**

  When used in combination with other antihypertensive medications, such as ACE inhibitors, ARBs (angiotensin receptor blockers), or calcium channel blockers, aldosterone antagonists can enhance the overall effectiveness of blood pressure management.

Heart Failure:

- **Role in Treatment:**

  In patients with heart failure, aldosterone contributes to sodium retention, fluid overload, and cardiac remodeling. By blocking aldosterone, these medications help reduce fluid retention, improve heart function, and prevent further damage to the heart.

- **Effectiveness:**

  Studies have shown that spironolactone and eplerenone reduce mortality in patients with heart failure, particularly those with **reduced ejection fraction** (HFrEF). Aldosterone antagonists are part of the standard treatment for heart failure, especially in patients with severe symptoms or who are hospitalized for heart failure exacerbations.

Chronic Kidney Disease (CKD) and Diabetic Nephropathy:

- **Role in Treatment:**

  In CKD, particularly in the context of **diabetic nephropathy** or **glomerulonephritis**, aldosterone promotes renal fibrosis, inflammation, and sodium retention. By blocking aldosterone, these medications help reduce proteinuria (excessive protein in the urine), which is a key marker of kidney damage.

- **Effectiveness:**

  Eplerenone and spironolactone are beneficial in slowing the progression of kidney disease by reducing inflammation and fibrosis. They are often used in patients with CKD who also have heart failure or hypertension.

Side Effects and Considerations in Treatment

While aldosterone antagonists are effective, they also come with certain side effects and considerations that must be carefully managed. Understanding these side effects is critical to ensuring the safe use of these medications.

1. **Hyperkalemia (High Potassium):**

Aldosterone antagonists promote potassium retention, which can lead to **hyperkalemia**. Elevated potassium levels can cause serious cardiac arrhythmias, muscle weakness, and other symptoms. Regular monitoring of potassium levels is essential, especially in patients with renal dysfunction, diabetes, or those on other medications that can increase potassium, such as ACE inhibitors or ARBs.

2. **Hypotension (Low Blood Pressure):**

Because aldosterone antagonists reduce blood volume, they can cause hypotension, particularly when starting treatment or increasing the dose. Patients should be monitored for symptoms of low blood pressure, such as dizziness, fainting, or lightheadedness, especially in the elderly or those with existing cardiovascular conditions.

3. **Hormonal Side Effects (Spironolactone):**

Spironolactone's non-selective inhibition of steroid receptors can lead to side effects related to its actions on androgens and progesterone. These include:

- **Gynecomastia (enlarged breasts in men)**
- **Menstrual irregularities** in women
- **Sexual dysfunction** (e.g., impotence in men)
- **Deepening of the voice** in women

4. Eplerenone, being more selective, tends to have fewer hormonal side effects, making it a better choice for patients at risk for these complications.

5. **Renal Function:**

Aldosterone antagonists can impact renal function, especially in patients with pre-existing kidney disease. Regular monitoring of kidney function (e.g., serum creatinine and glomerular filtration rate) is essential to ensure that renal function does not deteriorate with treatment.

6. **Drug Interactions:**

Both spironolactone and eplerenone can interact with other medications, including potassium supplements, ACE inhibitors, ARBs, and nonsteroidal anti-inflammatory drugs (NSAIDs). These interactions can increase the risk of hyperkalemia or exacerbate kidney function decline. Clinicians should review all medications a patient is taking to prevent adverse interactions.

Conclusion

Aldosterone antagonists, including spironolactone and eplerenone, have become an essential part of treatment regimens for conditions like hypertension, heart failure, and chronic kidney disease. By blocking aldosterone's effects on sodium retention and potassium excretion, these medications help reduce blood pressure, prevent fluid overload, and improve organ function. However, their use must be carefully monitored to avoid side effects like hyperkalemia and hypotension, and adjustments may be necessary based on individual patient needs.

As our understanding of aldosterone's role in various diseases continues to grow, the use of aldosterone antagonists is likely to expand, with new research focusing on their potential benefits in other conditions such as diabetes, stroke prevention, and fibrosis. The future of aldosterone-targeted therapies holds promise, with the possibility of even more effective and safer treatments for a range of cardiovascular, renal, and hormonal disorders.

Chapter 9: Aldosterone and Heart Health

Aldosterone, primarily known for its role in regulating fluid balance and blood pressure, also plays a critical role in cardiovascular health. Beyond its effect on the kidneys and electrolyte balance, aldosterone has significant implications for the heart, particularly in conditions such as heart failure, hypertension, and cardiovascular remodeling. This chapter explores how aldosterone influences heart health, the mechanisms through which it contributes to cardiac dysfunction, and how targeting aldosterone can improve outcomes in various cardiovascular conditions.

The Role of Aldosterone in Cardiovascular Disease

Aldosterone's effects on cardiovascular health go beyond simple regulation of blood pressure. It has been implicated in the pathophysiology of several cardiovascular diseases, particularly those associated with excessive aldosterone levels, such as **heart failure, hypertension**, and **cardiac fibrosis**. Understanding the role of aldosterone in these conditions is essential for managing cardiovascular disease and improving patient outcomes.

1. **Cardiac Remodeling:**

Aldosterone contributes to **cardiac remodeling**, a process in which the heart's structure and function change in response to chronic stress or injury. In heart failure, particularly with reduced ejection fraction (HFrEF), aldosterone's effects are amplified due to the activation of the renin-angiotensin-aldosterone system (RAAS). This leads to sodium and water retention, increased blood volume, and increased pressure on the heart. Over time, these changes lead to the thickening and stiffening of the heart's walls (fibrosis), which further impair its ability to pump effectively.

Aldosterone also promotes the accumulation of collagen in the myocardium (heart muscle), contributing to fibrosis. This can result in ventricular remodeling, where the heart's chambers enlarge, further weakening its pumping ability and increasing the risk of arrhythmias, heart failure exacerbations, and sudden cardiac death.

2. **Hypertension and Aldosterone:**

   Aldosterone is a major contributor to hypertension (high blood pressure),

   especially in individuals with **primary hyperaldosteronism** (Conn's syndrome),

   where aldosterone production is abnormally high. Elevated aldosterone levels lead

   to sodium retention, increased blood volume, and elevated vascular resistance, all

   of which contribute to sustained high blood pressure. Chronic hypertension

   increases the workload on the heart, causing damage to the blood vessels and the

   heart itself, potentially leading to stroke, kidney damage, and other complications.

   Furthermore, aldosterone's effects on vascular smooth muscle cells can increase

   vascular stiffness, which makes the heart work harder to pump blood throughout

   the body. This vascular remodeling, known as **arterial stiffness**, further elevates

   blood pressure and exacerbates cardiovascular strain.

Aldosterone's Impact on Cardiac Remodeling

Aldosterone's influence on cardiac remodeling is a key factor in the progression of heart

disease. Through its action on the heart and blood vessels, aldosterone promotes

processes that contribute to myocardial fibrosis, hypertrophy (abnormal enlargement of

heart cells), and electrical disturbances.

1. **Myocardial Fibrosis and Heart Failure:**

   In heart failure, aldosterone promotes the activation of fibroblasts, cells that produce collagen and other extracellular matrix components. This results in fibrosis within the myocardium, which leads to stiffening of the heart muscle, impaired ventricular filling, and decreased contractility. The fibrosis disrupts the normal architecture of the heart, making it less efficient and more prone to arrhythmias.

   This remodeling process is particularly pronounced in patients with **heart failure with reduced ejection fraction** (HFrEF), where the heart's ability to pump blood is compromised. Aldosterone's role in fibrosis makes it a key therapeutic target for heart failure treatment, as preventing or reversing fibrosis can help improve heart function and reduce the risk of hospitalization or death.

2. **Hypertrophy and Electrolyte Imbalance:**

   Aldosterone also promotes **cardiomyocyte hypertrophy**, the enlargement of individual heart muscle cells, as part of the remodeling process. Hypertrophic changes in the myocardium are often associated with increased stiffness, impaired relaxation, and diminished contractile function, which worsen heart failure. Additionally, aldosterone-induced **electrolyte imbalances**, particularly hypokalemia (low potassium) and hypernatremia (high sodium), contribute to arrhythmias and further impair heart function.

   Studies have shown that blocking aldosterone with **aldosterone antagonists**, such as spironolactone and eplerenone, can reduce myocardial fibrosis, prevent cardiac hypertrophy, and improve clinical outcomes in heart failure patients. These medications are considered a cornerstone of heart failure management, particularly in patients with reduced ejection fraction.

Targeting Aldosterone in Heart Failure Treatment

Given the substantial role that aldosterone plays in the progression of heart failure and other cardiovascular conditions, targeting aldosterone has become a key therapeutic strategy. The use of **aldosterone antagonists**—drugs that block the mineralocorticoid receptors in the heart, kidneys, and blood vessels—has proven to be effective in improving heart function, reducing symptoms, and prolonging life in heart failure patients.

1. **Spironolactone in Heart Failure:**

   Spironolactone has been extensively studied and shown to reduce mortality and morbidity in heart failure patients, particularly in those with **HFrEF**. By blocking aldosterone's effects on the heart, spironolactone reduces myocardial fibrosis, prevents arrhythmias, and decreases vascular resistance. The **RALES study** (Randomized Aldactone Evaluation Study) demonstrated that spironolactone significantly reduced the risk of death and hospitalization in patients with severe heart failure.

2. **Eplerenone in Heart Failure:**

   Eplerenone, a more selective aldosterone antagonist, has similar benefits to spironolactone but with a lower incidence of side effects, particularly those related to hormonal imbalance. The **EPHESUS trial** (Eplerenone Post-Acute Myocardial Infarction Heart Failure Efficacy and Survival Study) showed that eplerenone reduced mortality and hospitalizations in patients who had recently suffered a heart attack and had symptoms of heart failure or left ventricular dysfunction.

3. **Combined Therapy:**

In many cases, aldosterone antagonists are used in combination with other heart failure medications, such as **angiotensin-converting enzyme (ACE) inhibitors, angiotensin receptor blockers (ARBs)**, and **beta-blockers**. These combination therapies can provide additive benefits in reducing blood pressure, improving heart function, and reducing hospitalizations. The combination of an ACE inhibitor or ARB with an aldosterone antagonist is particularly effective in mitigating the harmful effects of aldosterone on the heart and kidneys.

Aldosterone and Other Cardiovascular Risk Factors

In addition to heart failure, aldosterone also plays a role in other cardiovascular diseases, such as **atrial fibrillation** (AF), **stroke**, and **coronary artery disease** (CAD). Its ability to promote sodium retention, vascular remodeling, and fibrosis contributes to an increased risk of these conditions. Moreover, aldosterone's effects on blood pressure and electrolyte balance make it a key factor in the development and progression of **hypertension**, which in turn increases the risk of stroke, heart attack, and kidney disease.

For patients with **atrial fibrillation**, aldosterone's role in promoting fibrosis in the atria may contribute to the electrical remodeling that underlies AF. In this context, aldosterone antagonists may offer benefits in reducing the incidence of AF and improving outcomes in patients with AF and heart failure.

Conclusion

Aldosterone's impact on cardiovascular health extends far beyond its role in regulating blood pressure and fluid balance. Through its effects on myocardial fibrosis, vascular remodeling, and electrolyte balance, aldosterone contributes to the progression of heart failure, hypertension, and other cardiovascular diseases. By targeting aldosterone with medications such as spironolactone and eplerenone, it is possible to reduce myocardial fibrosis, prevent arrhythmias, and improve heart function, thereby improving outcomes for patients with heart failure and other related conditions.

As research into aldosterone's role in cardiovascular disease continues, new therapies targeting aldosterone and its pathways hold promise for improving the treatment of heart failure, reducing the risk of stroke and heart attack, and enhancing overall cardiovascular health. Understanding the complex role of aldosterone in the cardiovascular system is crucial for optimizing treatment strategies and improving patient outcomes in cardiovascular disease.

Chapter 10: Aldosterone and the Kidneys

Aldosterone's impact on the kidneys is one of its most important roles in maintaining overall homeostasis. The kidneys regulate key functions such as fluid balance, blood pressure, and the excretion of metabolic waste. Aldosterone plays a pivotal role in modulating kidney function, particularly in the regulation of sodium, potassium, and water balance. This chapter explores how aldosterone affects renal function, its implications for kidney disease, and how therapies targeting aldosterone can improve outcomes in patients with renal disorders.

The Impact of Aldosterone on Renal Function

Aldosterone's primary action on the kidneys is through its effect on the distal tubules and collecting ducts. By binding to mineralocorticoid receptors, aldosterone influences the transport of sodium and potassium in the nephron. This effect is essential for regulating blood pressure, maintaining fluid balance, and ensuring electrolyte homeostasis.

1. **Sodium Reabsorption and Water Retention:** Aldosterone stimulates the reabsorption of sodium in the distal tubules and collecting ducts. This action directly influences the body's fluid balance because sodium, as a major extracellular cation, draws water back into the bloodstream. The reabsorption of sodium and water increases blood volume, thereby raising blood pressure. This process is crucial in maintaining normal blood pressure, particularly in response to blood loss, dehydration, or low blood sodium levels.

2. **Potassium Excretion:** One of the key roles of aldosterone in the kidneys is to regulate potassium levels. As sodium is reabsorbed, potassium is excreted into the urine in a process called **potassium secretion**. Aldosterone promotes this exchange by stimulating sodium-potassium pumps, which move sodium from the tubule lumen back into the bloodstream and potassium into the tubular lumen for excretion. Maintaining the right balance of sodium and potassium is critical for normal cell function, nerve conduction, and muscle contraction.

3. **Acid-Base Balance:** Aldosterone also plays a role in maintaining acid-base balance. In the kidneys, it promotes the exchange of sodium for hydrogen ions in the tubules. This helps to regulate the pH of the blood by reducing the acidity, which is particularly important during times of metabolic acidosis.

By coordinating sodium, potassium, and water balance, aldosterone ensures proper kidney function and contributes to systemic homeostasis. When aldosterone levels are dysregulated, it can lead to a variety of renal and systemic complications.

Aldosterone in Kidney Disease and Dialysis

Chronic kidney disease (CKD) and acute kidney injury (AKI) can significantly alter the normal regulation of aldosterone, with both increased and decreased secretion being implicated in kidney dysfunction.

1. **Hyperaldosteronism and Kidney Disease:** In conditions such as **primary hyperaldosteronism** (Conn's syndrome), where aldosterone is overproduced, excessive sodium and water retention can worsen kidney disease by increasing blood pressure and contributing to further glomerular injury. Hyperaldosteronism is associated with **proteinuria** (protein in the urine), which is a hallmark of kidney damage. The excess sodium and water burden also increase the workload on the kidneys, contributing to glomerulosclerosis (scarring of the kidney's filtering units) and ultimately leading to kidney failure.

2. **Aldosterone and Kidney Fibrosis:** Aldosterone has been shown to promote kidney fibrosis by activating fibroblasts, which deposit collagen and other extracellular matrix components. This fibrosis contributes to the progressive loss of kidney function. In conditions like diabetic nephropathy, hypertension, and glomerulonephritis, excessive aldosterone accelerates kidney damage through these mechanisms.

3. **Aldosterone Antagonists in Renal Disease:** The use of aldosterone antagonists, such as **spironolactone** and **eplerenone**, has proven beneficial in managing kidney disease, particularly in cases of **heart failure** and **diabetic nephropathy**. These medications help reduce proteinuria, preserve kidney function, and prevent further damage to the glomeruli. By blocking aldosterone, these drugs prevent sodium retention and reduce the risk of fibrosis and scarring in the kidneys. Additionally, they may improve vascular function and lower blood pressure, further benefiting kidney health.

- **Spironolactone:** In patients with CKD, particularly those with heart failure, spironolactone has been shown to reduce the risk of progression to end-stage renal disease (ESRD). Spironolactone's ability to decrease proteinuria and lower blood pressure makes it a valuable addition to treatment regimens aimed at slowing kidney deterioration.

- **Eplerenone:** A more selective aldosterone antagonist, eplerenone is less likely to cause side effects related to hormonal imbalances and is typically used in cases where spironolactone's side effects are problematic. Eplerenone's role in treating CKD and preventing further kidney damage is supported by studies demonstrating its efficacy in reducing proteinuria and improving kidney function.

Dialysis and Aldosterone:

Therapeutic Approaches in Renal Disorders

Effective management of aldosterone's effects on kidney function involves a combination of pharmacological and non-pharmacological approaches. These therapies aim to balance aldosterone levels, improve kidney health, and prevent further complications.

1. **Aldosterone Antagonists in Renal Disease Management:** As mentioned, aldosterone antagonists such as spironolactone and eplerenone play a key role in managing CKD, particularly in patients with associated heart failure or hypertension. These drugs should be used carefully, with close monitoring of potassium levels, kidney function, and blood pressure.

2. **Angiotensin Converting Enzyme (ACE) Inhibitors and ARBs:** ACE inhibitors and angiotensin receptor blockers (ARBs) are commonly used in kidney disease, particularly in patients with proteinuria. These medications reduce the activation of the RAAS and lower aldosterone secretion, helping to protect the kidneys from further damage. ACE inhibitors and ARBs work synergistically with aldosterone antagonists to slow the progression of kidney disease.

3. **Dietary Modifications:** A balanced diet is an important component of kidney disease management. Reducing dietary sodium intake helps to reduce fluid retention and manage blood pressure. Potassium levels should also be monitored, as both high and low potassium levels can be harmful, especially in patients with kidney dysfunction.

4. **Blood Pressure Control:** Blood pressure management is crucial in preventing further kidney damage. In CKD patients, maintaining a target blood pressure
Conclusion
(typically less than 130/80 mm Hg) helps prevent the progression of renal damage and reduces the risk of cardiovascular complications.

Aldosterone plays a vital role in kidney function, regulating sodium, potassium, and fluid balance. Dysregulation of aldosterone, whether through overproduction or insufficient production, can lead to significant kidney damage and worsen conditions such as hypertension, heart failure, and chronic kidney disease. Aldosterone antagonists have become an essential tool in managing kidney disease, particularly in preventing fibrosis, reducing proteinuria, and preserving kidney function. Through careful management of aldosterone levels and appropriate pharmacological interventions, it is possible to slow the progression of kidney disease and improve long-term outcomes. As research into aldosterone's role in kidney health continues, new therapeutic approaches and drug formulations may provide even more effective ways to protect and enhance renal function.

Chapter 11: Aldosterone and the Brain

Aldosterone, while primarily known for its effects on the kidneys and cardiovascular system, also exerts significant influence on the brain. This influence goes beyond its role in fluid balance and blood pressure regulation and extends to neurovascular health, cognition, stress responses, and the modulation of behaviors. In this chapter, we will explore how aldosterone affects brain function, its potential link to neurological disorders, and the emerging understanding of aldosterone's role in modulating neurovascular health and stress responses.

How Aldosterone Affects Neurovascular Health

The brain relies heavily on a delicate balance of electrolytes, hydration, and blood flow to maintain normal function. Aldosterone plays a crucial role in regulating this balance by influencing both the **cerebral vasculature** (the blood vessels supplying the brain) and **electrolyte levels** that are important for neuronal activity.

1. **Blood Pressure and Cerebral Blood Flow:** Aldosterone's regulation of blood pressure indirectly affects cerebral blood flow (CBF). The hormone's impact on vascular tone, particularly in the arteries, can influence the amount of blood that reaches the brain. Elevated aldosterone levels lead to increased vascular resistance, which raises blood pressure. While this is crucial for maintaining adequate perfusion to various organs, excessive aldosterone can cause **hypertension**, which is a known risk factor for stroke and other neurovascular diseases. Chronic hypertension can result in **vascular remodeling**, which increases the risk of blood-brain barrier dysfunction, cerebral edema, and hemorrhagic stroke.

   By controlling vascular tone, aldosterone plays a direct role in regulating CBF, ensuring the brain receives an adequate supply of oxygenated blood. However, in excess, aldosterone may contribute to the pathogenesis of cerebrovascular disorders through persistent vascular constriction and damage.

2. **Blood-Brain Barrier Integrity:** The blood-brain barrier (BBB) is a selective permeability barrier that regulates the entry of ions, molecules, and pathogens into the brain. Aldosterone, through its influence on blood pressure and vascular tone, may impact the integrity of this barrier. Some studies suggest that elevated aldosterone levels can increase **vascular permeability**, potentially leading to leakage of harmful substances into the brain and exacerbating neuroinflammation. This effect has been linked to neurodegenerative diseases such as Alzheimer's and cognitive decline.

The Role of Aldosterone in Brain Function and Stroke Risk

Aldosterone's direct effects on the brain are most notable in its interaction with the **central nervous system (CNS),** particularly in the regulation of **cognition, stress responses,** and **neuroinflammation.**

1. **Aldosterone and Cognitive Function:** Research has shown that aldosterone may influence cognitive performance through its action on the hippocampus, a brain region essential for memory and learning. In particular, aldosterone appears to modulate **synaptic plasticity**, the ability of neurons to strengthen or weaken their connections in response to stimuli. This process is vital for memory formation and cognitive function. Disruption of aldosterone signaling may impair synaptic plasticity, potentially contributing to cognitive decline seen in diseases such as Alzheimer's disease and other forms of dementia.

2. **Aldosterone as a Modulator of Stroke Risk:** Aldosterone's effect on vascular health has implications for the risk of **ischemic stroke** (due to lack of blood supply to the brain) and **hemorrhagic stroke** (due to blood vessel rupture). Chronic high blood pressure, often driven by excessive aldosterone, is a primary risk factor for stroke. Aldosterone's role in promoting vascular damage and fluid retention can increase the likelihood of cerebrovascular events. By encouraging vascular fibrosis and endothelial dysfunction, aldosterone may contribute to a more rigid and less responsive vascular system, thereby increasing the risk of atherosclerosis and clot formation.

3. **Neuroinflammation and Aldosterone:** High aldosterone levels may also be involved in **neuroinflammation**, a process linked to many neurological diseases. Neuroinflammation involves the activation of glial cells, such as microglia, which release inflammatory cytokines in response to injury or disease. Chronic activation of these cells can contribute to neuronal damage and neurodegeneration. Studies suggest that aldosterone may contribute to the activation of microglia and the subsequent release of pro-inflammatory cytokines, exacerbating neuroinflammatory conditions such as Alzheimer's, Parkinson's, and multiple sclerosis.

Aldosterone as a Modulator of Stress Responses

Aldosterone is closely tied to the body's response to stress through its interactions with the **hypothalamic-pituitary-adrenal (HPA) axis**, which regulates the release of cortisol and other stress-related hormones. This connection is crucial for understanding how aldosterone may influence mood, behavior, and stress management.

1. **Aldosterone and the HPA Axis:** The HPA axis is responsible for the body's physiological response to stress, involving the release of cortisol from the adrenal glands. When stress occurs, aldosterone levels typically increase to help manage the fluid balance and blood pressure response. The relationship between aldosterone and cortisol is bidirectional: cortisol can influence aldosterone secretion, and aldosterone can enhance the effects of cortisol. When this system is dysregulated—such as in chronic stress, anxiety, or mood disorders—elevated aldosterone may exacerbate the negative effects of chronic cortisol elevation, such as hypertension, sleep disturbances, and heightened anxiety.

2. **Mood Disorders and Stress Resilience:** Elevated aldosterone may impair the body's ability to cope with stress effectively. In animal models, increased aldosterone levels have been associated with heightened anxiety-like behaviors, potentially due to the hormone's impact on brain regions involved in emotional regulation, such as the prefrontal cortex and amygdala. In humans, chronic stress and the associated activation of the RAAS system may contribute to mood disorders such as **depression** and **generalized anxiety disorder**. By regulating aldosterone, it may be possible to improve stress resilience and reduce the psychological burden associated with chronic stress.

Aldosterone and Electrolyte Imbalance in the Brain

The balance of electrolytes such as sodium and potassium is essential not only for kidney function and blood pressure regulation but also for **neuronal excitability** and **synaptic function** in the brain. Aldosterone's role in maintaining this balance can have direct implications for brain function.

1. **Sodium and Potassium in Neuronal Activity:** Neurons rely on a delicate balance of sodium and potassium gradients across their membranes to generate action potentials, which are the electrical signals that allow communication between nerve cells. Aldosterone's role in regulating sodium reabsorption and potassium excretion can influence neuronal activity. An imbalance in these ions can lead to altered neuronal firing patterns, which can impact cognition, mood, and overall brain function. In conditions such as **hypokalemia** (low potassium) or **hypernatremia** (high sodium), the resulting electrolyte disturbances can lead to symptoms such as confusion, seizures, and cognitive dysfunction.

2. **Neurological Implications of Electrolyte Imbalance:** Long-term aldosterone dysregulation can lead to sustained electrolyte imbalances, which are associated with a variety of neurological disorders. For example, **hyponatremia** (low sodium) has been linked to confusion and delirium, particularly in elderly patients. **Hyperkalemia** (high potassium), often a consequence of aldosterone antagonists or adrenal insufficiency, can lead to dangerous arrhythmias and even cardiac arrest, both of which have direct implications for brain function due to lack of oxygen and perfusion.

Conclusion

Aldosterone's influence extends far beyond its traditional roles in the kidneys and cardiovascular system. Through its effects on neurovascular health, cognition, stress responses, and electrolyte balance, aldosterone plays a key role in brain function. Dysregulated aldosterone levels can contribute to a variety of neurological disorders, including stroke, cognitive decline, mood disorders, and neuroinflammation.

Understanding the complex interactions between aldosterone and the brain opens new avenues for therapeutic interventions targeting this hormone in conditions such as Alzheimer's disease, depression, and stroke. With ongoing research into the role of aldosterone in neurovascular health, future therapies may aim to modulate aldosterone signaling to protect and enhance brain function, ultimately leading to better outcomes for individuals with neurological conditions and those at risk for cerebrovascular events.

Chapter 12: Measuring Aldosterone Levels

Accurately measuring aldosterone levels is crucial for diagnosing and managing disorders related to aldosterone dysregulation. Given aldosterone's significant role in blood pressure regulation, electrolyte balance, and fluid homeostasis, its measurement can provide essential insights into various medical conditions, such as **hypertension**, **heart failure**, **kidney disease**, and **endocrine disorders**. In this chapter, we will explore the different methods used to measure aldosterone levels, the interpretation of test results, and the challenges associated with accurate diagnosis. Additionally, we will discuss the clinical applications and diagnostic challenges when assessing aldosterone.

Blood Tests and Urinary Tests for Aldosterone Levels

There are two primary methods for assessing aldosterone levels: **serum (blood) tests** and **urinary tests**. Each has its specific applications and advantages, and their use depends on the clinical situation.

Serum Aldosterone Measurement:

serum blood tests

primary aldosteronism

secondary hyperaldosteronism

aldosterone deficiency

Procedure:

supine (lying down)

upright (standing)

- **Normal Reference Ranges:**
  Normal aldosterone levels in the blood vary by lab, but a typical reference range is **3-16 ng/dL** in the upright position and **1-6 ng/dL** when lying down. These values may differ based on factors like time of day, age, and sex.
- **Conditions Indicated by Serum Aldosterone Testing:**
- **Primary Aldosteronism (Conn's Syndrome):** Elevated aldosterone with low renin levels in the blood.
- **Secondary Hyperaldosteronism:** Elevated aldosterone with elevated renin levels due to conditions like **renal artery stenosis** or **heart failure**.
- **Aldosterone Deficiency:** Low aldosterone levels, which could be indicative of conditions like **Addison's disease**.

Urinary Aldosterone Measurement:

- **Procedure:**

  A 24-hour urine collection is performed to capture the full spectrum of aldosterone excretion over a 24-hour period. This method is used for more detailed assessments of aldosterone production, as it averages out fluctuations in secretion over the course of the day.

- **Conditions Indicated by Urinary Aldosterone Testing:**

- **Hypertension:** If aldosterone levels are high in urine, it may suggest overproduction or underutilization of aldosterone by the kidneys.

- **Renal Dysfunction:** Changes in aldosterone excretion can help assess kidney function, especially in patients with suspected **renal artery stenosis** or **chronic kidney disease**.

Aldosterone-to-Renin Ratio (ARR):

aldosterone-to-renin ratio (ARR)

- **Procedure:**

  The ARR is typically calculated from serum samples, with aldosterone and renin levels measured simultaneously. A high ARR suggests **primary aldosteronism**, as aldosterone is elevated while renin is low, indicating autonomous production of aldosterone by the adrenal glands.

- **Conditions Indicated by ARR Testing:**

- **Primary Aldosteronism:** The hallmark of this condition is an elevated aldosterone-to-renin ratio, suggesting that the adrenal glands are producing aldosterone independent of renin.

- **Essential Hypertension:** If both aldosterone and renin levels are low, it may indicate essential hypertension, which is not linked to aldosterone overproduction.

Interpreting Test Results

Interpreting aldosterone levels requires careful consideration of the clinical context, including the patient's medical history, symptoms, and the presence of other comorbidities. Several factors can influence aldosterone levels, making interpretation challenging.

Physiological Variations:

- **Posture:** As mentioned earlier, the patient's position during testing can significantly affect aldosterone levels. This is why standardization is crucial for accurate results.

- **Time of Day:** Aldosterone levels typically follow a circadian rhythm, with the highest levels occurring in the early morning and the lowest in the evening.

- **Diet:** High sodium intake can suppress aldosterone levels, while low sodium intake can stimulate aldosterone production. A high-potassium diet can also increase aldosterone secretion.

Medications and Treatments:

ACE inhibitors

angiotensin receptor blockers (ARBs)

diuretics

beta-blockers

- **Aldosterone Antagonists (Spironolactone, Eplerenone):** These medications block aldosterone's effects, so they can alter both serum and urinary aldosterone levels. Patients taking these drugs may need to be off them for a period before testing.
- **Diuretics:** These medications, especially potassium-sparing diuretics, can affect aldosterone secretion and electrolyte balance, complicating the interpretation of results.
- **Steroid Medications:** Corticosteroids can also influence aldosterone production by mimicking aldosterone's effects on sodium and fluid retention.

Diagnostic Challenges and Solutions:

primary aldosteronism

- **Fludrocortisone suppression test:** This test involves administering a synthetic steroid to suppress aldosterone production. A failure to suppress aldosterone is indicative of primary aldosteronism.
- **Saline infusion test:** This test involves infusing saline into the patient's bloodstream to suppress aldosterone secretion. An inadequate response suggests aldosterone overproduction.

Clinical Applications of Aldosterone Measurement

The measurement of aldosterone levels is essential for diagnosing and managing various medical conditions. Key clinical applications include:

Hypertension Management:

- Measuring aldosterone levels helps to diagnose secondary causes of hypertension, such as **primary aldosteronism, renal artery stenosis**, or **Cushing's syndrome.** Early identification of these causes can lead to more targeted and effective treatment strategies.
- For resistant hypertension (cases where blood pressure does not respond to multiple medications), measuring aldosterone and renin levels can guide appropriate therapy.

Heart Failure:

Aldosterone measurement is essential in evaluating

 patients, particularly those with

. Elevated aldosterone levels are often present in heart failure due to fluid retention, and aldosterone antagonists like spironolactone and eplerenone are crucial for managing these patients.

Kidney Disease:

Measuring aldosterone levels is vital for assessing patients with

,

, or

. Aldosterone contributes to kidney fibrosis and proteinuria, so monitoring its levels helps in evaluating disease progression and the effectiveness of therapy.

Endocrine Disorders:

Testing aldosterone levels is crucial for diagnosing conditions like

(aldosterone deficiency) and

(excessive aldosterone production). Correct diagnosis and treatment are essential for managing these endocrine disorders effectively.

Conclusion

Measuring aldosterone levels is a powerful tool in diagnosing and managing various conditions, particularly those related to blood pressure, heart failure, kidney disease, and endocrine dysfunction. Accurate testing, careful interpretation of results, and awareness of physiological and medication-induced factors are essential for proper diagnosis and treatment. As research continues into the role of aldosterone in health and disease, advancements in testing methods and therapeutic strategies will further enhance our ability to manage aldosterone-related disorders and optimize patient care.

Chapter 13: Aldosterone and Cancer

Aldosterone, primarily known for its role in regulating blood pressure, fluid balance, and electrolyte levels, has recently been implicated in the pathophysiology of cancer. While much of the research on aldosterone has focused on its cardiovascular and renal effects, emerging evidence suggests that this hormone may also play a significant role in the development and progression of various cancers. In this chapter, we will explore the potential link between aldosterone and cancer, how aldosterone may influence tumor growth, and the possibility of targeting aldosterone in cancer therapy. We will also discuss lifestyle modifications that may help optimize aldosterone function and reduce cancer risk.

Exploring the Link Between Aldosterone and Cancer Risk

Recent studies have suggested that aldosterone may contribute to the development and progression of cancer through several mechanisms, including inflammation, oxidative stress, and tissue remodeling. These effects are particularly relevant in cancers that are associated with high levels of aldosterone, such as breast, prostate, and colon cancers.

Aldosterone and Tumor Growth:

- **Proliferation and Metastasis:**

  Aldosterone has been shown to influence cellular processes that are crucial for tumor growth, including cell proliferation, apoptosis (cell death), and migration. It is believed that aldosterone can activate signaling pathways that promote the growth and spread of cancer cells. The mineralocorticoid receptor (MR), which aldosterone binds to, is present not only in the kidneys and heart but also in various tissues, including the **epithelial cells** in the breast, prostate, and colon. When aldosterone binds to these receptors, it can trigger a cascade of events that enhance cancer cell proliferation and metastasis.

- **Angiogenesis:**

  Aldosterone has been implicated in **angiogenesis**, the formation of new blood vessels, which is essential for tumor growth. Tumors require a blood supply to grow and metastasize, and aldosterone may contribute to this process by increasing the production of angiogenic factors like **vascular endothelial growth factor (VEGF)**. This promotes the growth of blood vessels that nourish tumors, enabling them to expand and invade surrounding tissues.

2. **Inflammation and Immune Response:** Chronic inflammation is a well-known risk factor for cancer, and aldosterone may exacerbate this by promoting an inflammatory environment in tissues. Aldosterone can stimulate the production of pro-inflammatory cytokines and activate immune cells such as **macrophages** and **T-cells**, which may contribute to tumor growth and metastasis. Additionally, aldosterone may influence the **tumor microenvironment**, a complex network of cells and molecules surrounding a tumor that plays a key role in tumor progression and resistance to therapy.

   The presence of **fibroblasts** (cells that produce collagen and other extracellular matrix components) in the tumor microenvironment is also influenced by aldosterone. These fibroblasts contribute to fibrosis (the thickening and scarring of tissue) and can promote the progression of certain types of cancer, particularly in the **liver** and **lung**. Aldosterone's role in fibrosis may therefore contribute to the growth and spread of cancer cells.

3. **Oxidative Stress:** Aldosterone is also thought to contribute to **oxidative stress**, a condition characterized by the excessive production of reactive oxygen species (ROS), which can damage cells and lead to mutations. High aldosterone levels may increase oxidative stress in tissues, further promoting cellular changes that lead to cancerous transformation. Oxidative stress has been implicated in several types of cancer, and aldosterone's role in this process highlights its potential impact on cancer risk and progression.

4. **Aldosterone, Obesity, and Cancer:** Research has suggested that obesity, which is associated with increased aldosterone levels, may increase the risk of several types of cancer, including **breast cancer, endometrial cancer**, and **colorectal cancer**. In obese individuals, elevated aldosterone levels may contribute to insulin resistance, chronic inflammation, and altered cell signaling, all of which are linked to an increased cancer risk. Addressing aldosterone levels in obese patients may help mitigate this risk and reduce the likelihood of developing cancer.

How Aldosterone May Influence Tumor Growth

The mechanisms through which aldosterone influences tumor growth are multifaceted and still being explored. Some of the most prominent ways aldosterone contributes to cancer development and progression include:

1. **Mineralocorticoid Receptor (MR) Activation:** Aldosterone's binding to mineralocorticoid receptors (MR) on target cells is key to its action in promoting cancer cell proliferation. MR activation triggers intracellular signaling pathways that regulate gene expression related to cell growth, migration, and survival. For example, aldosterone has been shown to activate the **PI3K/Akt** pathway, which is involved in cell survival, and the **MAPK** pathway, which regulates cell proliferation. By modulating these pathways, aldosterone may promote the growth and spread of cancer cells.

2. **Fibrosis and Tissue Remodeling:** Fibrosis is a key feature of many types of cancer, and aldosterone contributes to this process by promoting the activation of fibroblasts, which in turn produce collagen and other extracellular matrix components. This process can create a supportive environment for tumor growth and invasion, allowing cancer cells to spread to other parts of the body.

3. **Interaction with Angiotensin II:** Aldosterone often works in tandem with **angiotensin II**, another key component of the RAAS system. Angiotensin II is known to stimulate blood vessel constriction and increase blood pressure, both of which are important for sustaining tumor growth. Aldosterone can enhance the effects of angiotensin II, further promoting tumor growth through increased blood flow and angiogenesis.

4. **Epithelial-Mesenchymal Transition (EMT):** Aldosterone may play a role in **epithelial-mesenchymal transition (EMT)**, a process that allows epithelial cells (cells that line organs) to become more migratory and invasive, facilitating cancer metastasis. EMT is a critical step in the spread of many cancers, and aldosterone may facilitate this transition by promoting changes in cell structure and function.

Targeting Aldosterone in Cancer Therapy

Given its potential role in promoting tumor growth, aldosterone represents an attractive target for cancer therapy. Research into **aldosterone antagonists**, such as spironolactone and eplerenone, has suggested that these drugs may have potential therapeutic benefits in cancer treatment.

1. **Aldosterone Antagonists as Cancer Therapies:** Aldosterone antagonists, by blocking the action of aldosterone at the mineralocorticoid receptor, may help reduce cancer cell proliferation, angiogenesis, and metastasis. Although primarily used in conditions like heart failure and hypertension, these medications may be repurposed for cancer therapy. Some studies have shown that spironolactone can inhibit the growth of certain cancer cell lines, particularly in **breast cancer** and **prostate cancer**, by reducing aldosterone's effects on cell proliferation and inflammation.

2. **Combination Therapy:** Aldosterone antagonists may be most effective when used in combination with other cancer treatments, such as chemotherapy, radiation therapy, or targeted therapies. Combining aldosterone blockers with drugs that inhibit the RAAS system could enhance the therapeutic effects by reducing the tumor's blood supply and inhibiting cancer cell growth and survival. Research into combination therapies involving aldosterone antagonists is ongoing, and early results are promising.

3. **Selective Targeting:** Research is also focused on developing more selective mineralocorticoid receptor antagonists or inhibitors that specifically target aldosterone's effects on tumor cells without causing unwanted side effects. By

Lifestyle Modifications for Optimizing Aldosterone Function

selectively targeting the pathways involved in tumor growth, these treatments could offer a more precise approach to cancer therapy.

Given aldosterone's potential role in cancer, managing its levels through lifestyle modifications may reduce cancer risk and improve overall health.

1. **Reducing Stress:**

   Chronic stress can lead to the activation of the HPA axis and RAAS system, increasing aldosterone levels. Engaging in stress-reducing activities such as mindfulness, yoga, deep breathing, and regular physical exercise may help maintain balanced aldosterone levels and reduce cancer risk.

2. **Diet and Nutrition:**

   A diet rich in fruits, vegetables, and antioxidants may help reduce oxidative stress and inflammation, both of which are implicated in cancer development. Limiting salt intake can also help manage aldosterone levels, as high sodium intake can stimulate aldosterone production.

3. **Regular Exercise:**

   Regular physical activity is known to reduce aldosterone levels by improving cardiovascular function, reducing inflammation, and promoting hormonal balance. Exercise may also enhance the effectiveness of cancer treatments and reduce the risk of recurrence in cancer survivors.

Conclusion

The emerging evidence linking aldosterone to cancer underscores the need for a deeper understanding of how this hormone influences tumor biology. While much of the research is still in its early stages, targeting aldosterone in cancer therapy presents an exciting avenue for improving treatment outcomes. Furthermore, managing aldosterone levels through lifestyle modifications, stress reduction, and proper diet may help reduce cancer risk and promote overall health. As research continues to evolve, aldosterone may become an increasingly important target in the fight against cancer.

Chapter 15: Stress Reduction and Its Effect on Aldosterone

Aldosterone is a key hormone in regulating blood pressure, fluid balance, and electrolyte homeostasis. However, its secretion can be influenced by various factors, one of the most significant being **stress**. Stress activates the body's physiological response mechanisms, including the **hypothalamic-pituitary-adrenal (HPA) axis** and the **renin-angiotensin-aldosterone system (RAAS)**. Over time, chronic stress can lead to dysregulated aldosterone levels, contributing to health conditions such as hypertension, cardiovascular disease, and kidney dysfunction. This chapter explores the relationship between stress and aldosterone, how stress management techniques can help optimize aldosterone function, and the potential benefits of reducing stress for overall health and well-being.

The Interplay Between Stress and Aldosterone

1. **Activation of the HPA Axis and RAAS:** Stress triggers the activation of the **HPA axis**, which leads to the release of cortisol, the body's primary stress hormone. Cortisol, in turn, influences aldosterone secretion. Stress also activates the **RAAS**, further promoting aldosterone release. When the body experiences physical or emotional stress, this cascade of hormonal responses serves to prepare the body to respond to perceived threats—commonly referred to as the "fight or flight" response. Aldosterone's role in this response is to ensure the retention of sodium and water, thereby increasing blood volume and maintaining blood pressure.

2. **Chronic Stress and Aldosterone Dysregulation:** While short-term stress responses are adaptive and necessary for survival, chronic stress can lead to sustained high levels of cortisol and aldosterone. Elevated cortisol levels from prolonged stress can promote aldosterone production and contribute to **fluid retention, increased blood pressure**, and **electrolyte imbalances**. Over time, this chronic activation of both the HPA axis and RAAS can have negative consequences on cardiovascular health, kidney function, and overall metabolic regulation. Prolonged stress-induced aldosterone release can contribute to conditions such as **hypertension, heart disease, stroke**, and **kidney disease**.

The Effects of Chronic Stress on Blood Pressure and Health

Chronic stress not only leads to sustained high aldosterone levels but also impacts blood pressure regulation. Elevated aldosterone levels in response to stress increase sodium retention, resulting in **water retention** and **increased blood volume**. This can lead to **elevated blood pressure**, a condition known as **stress-induced hypertension**. Over time, the continued elevation in blood pressure may contribute to the development of **cardiovascular disease**, including **arterial stiffness**, **heart failure**, and **kidney damage**.

Furthermore, the combination of stress-induced aldosterone release and the **sympathetic nervous system activation**—which also occurs during stress—can worsen the effects of hypertension. The sympathetic nervous system increases heart rate and blood vessel constriction, while aldosterone exacerbates sodium and fluid retention, creating a vicious cycle that further elevates blood pressure. This cycle can increase the workload on the heart, promote arterial damage, and increase the risk of **stroke** and **heart attacks**.

Stress and the Impact on Kidney Function

The kidneys are heavily influenced by aldosterone, as it regulates sodium, potassium, and fluid balance. Chronic stress-induced aldosterone secretion can increase the workload on the kidneys, contributing to **kidney dysfunction** and **proteinuria** (protein in the urine). Over time, the persistent elevation of aldosterone, along with the negative impact of high blood pressure on the kidneys, can result in **chronic kidney disease (CKD)**. Managing stress and optimizing aldosterone levels may play a key role in preventing the progression of kidney disease and maintaining kidney health.

Stress Reduction Techniques and Their Impact on Aldosterone Levels

Given the impact of chronic stress on aldosterone secretion and overall health, stress reduction techniques are essential for restoring hormonal balance and improving well-being. The following methods have been shown to help regulate stress and aldosterone levels:

Mindfulness and Meditation:

Breathing exercises:

Physical Exercise:

- **Aerobic exercise** (such as walking, running, or swimming) and **strength training** can help regulate aldosterone levels by improving blood circulation, enhancing kidney function, and reducing blood pressure.

- **Yoga and Tai Chi**: These practices combine physical movement with deep breathing and mindfulness, which can help reduce cortisol and aldosterone levels while promoting relaxation and overall mental well-being.

Adequate Sleep:

Aim for

per night to allow for the body's natural processes of healing and hormonal regulation. Improving sleep hygiene, such as maintaining a consistent sleep schedule, limiting screen time before bed, and creating a calm sleep environment, can help promote better rest and reduce stress.

4. **Social Support and Stress Management:** Strong social connections and a support network are essential for managing stress. Studies have shown that social interactions can reduce the physiological impacts of stress and help lower cortisol levels. Talking to friends, family, or a mental health professional can provide emotional support and help alleviate stress. Engaging in social activities or joining support groups can also improve overall well-being.

5. **Cognitive Behavioral Therapy (CBT):** Cognitive behavioral therapy is an evidence-based treatment designed to help individuals manage stress, anxiety, and depression. CBT helps patients identify and reframe negative thought patterns that contribute to stress and emotional distress. This therapy has been shown to reduce cortisol levels and improve psychological well-being, leading to better hormonal balance and reduced aldosterone secretion.

Diet and Hydration: Supporting Stress Reduction and Aldosterone Balance

Diet plays a crucial role in managing stress and optimizing aldosterone function. Proper nutrition can reduce inflammation, improve cardiovascular health, and support adrenal function, which is essential for managing stress.

Reducing Sodium Intake:

Recommendations:

DASH diet

2. **Incorporating Potassium-Rich Foods:** Potassium helps balance the effects of sodium in the body and supports healthy kidney function. Foods rich in potassium, such as **bananas**, **avocados**, **sweet potatoes**, and **leafy greens**, can help manage aldosterone-induced imbalances and promote fluid balance.

3. **Adequate Hydration:** Proper hydration is essential for maintaining aldosterone balance. Dehydration can trigger aldosterone secretion to conserve water, while overhydration can suppress aldosterone release. Drinking enough water throughout the day helps maintain fluid balance and supports kidney function.

Conclusion

Chronic stress can lead to dysregulated aldosterone secretion, contributing to a range of health issues such as hypertension, kidney disease, and cardiovascular dysfunction. By implementing effective stress reduction techniques, such as mindfulness, exercise, and proper sleep, individuals can help optimize aldosterone function and reduce the negative impact of stress on overall health. A holistic approach that includes dietary modifications, social support, and psychological well-being can further enhance stress management and improve long-term health outcomes. Through mastering stress and understanding its effects on aldosterone, we can create a foundation for better health, vitality, and longevity.

Chapter 16: Aldosterone and Aging

As we age, the body undergoes a series of physiological changes that affect various systems, including the hormonal systems that regulate critical processes such as fluid balance, blood pressure, and electrolyte homeostasis. Aldosterone, a hormone primarily responsible for regulating sodium and water balance, plays a crucial role in maintaining these processes. However, aging can impact aldosterone secretion, its effectiveness, and its interactions with other hormones, contributing to age-related health conditions. In this chapter, we will explore how aging affects aldosterone secretion, its relationship to the aging cardiovascular system, and the impact of aldosterone imbalances in older adults. We will also discuss strategies for managing aldosterone levels to improve overall health in the aging population.

How Aging Affects Aldosterone Secretion

Aldosterone secretion follows a circadian rhythm, with levels typically peaking in the morning and declining throughout the day. This pattern can be altered with age. Research suggests that **aging** can lead to **altered aldosterone production**, with some older adults experiencing a decrease in aldosterone responsiveness. The following factors are thought to contribute to changes in aldosterone secretion with age:

1. **Reduced Renal Function:** The kidneys play a central role in aldosterone regulation. As people age, kidney function naturally declines, leading to a reduced ability to filter blood, balance electrolytes, and regulate fluid levels. This decreased renal function can impair the kidney's ability to respond to aldosterone, resulting in **increased aldosterone production** or impaired **aldosterone clearance** from the body. This contributes to an imbalance in fluid regulation, often manifesting as **hypertension** or **edema** in older adults.

2. **Decreased Renin-Angiotensin-Aldosterone System (RAAS) Activity:** The RAAS system is the primary pathway responsible for aldosterone secretion. Studies have shown that while **renin** levels tend to decrease with age, aldosterone secretion can still remain relatively high due to increased sodium retention in the kidneys. However, this imbalance can make it harder for the body to adjust fluid and sodium balance in response to various physiological changes, increasing the risk of both **high blood pressure** and **fluid retention** in the elderly.

3. **Changes in Mineralocorticoid Receptor Sensitivity:** The sensitivity of **mineralocorticoid receptors** (MRs) to aldosterone may also decrease with age. MRs are found in tissues such as the kidneys, heart, and brain, where aldosterone exerts its effects. As people age, a **diminished sensitivity** of these receptors can reduce the efficiency of aldosterone in promoting sodium reabsorption, potentially resulting in **impaired fluid balance** and contributing to the development of **hypertension** or **hypotension**.

4. **Decline in Cortisol Secretion:** As the body ages, cortisol production, which is linked to aldosterone through the **HPA axis**, may decline. This reduction in cortisol may affect aldosterone's balance with other hormones and influence its activity in ways that can contribute to **hypertension** and other age-related health conditions.

Aldosterone and the Aging Cardiovascular System

The aging cardiovascular system is particularly vulnerable to aldosterone imbalances. As aldosterone continues to influence sodium and water retention, its effects on blood pressure regulation become more pronounced in older adults. Aging leads to several changes in the cardiovascular system, including increased vascular stiffness, endothelial dysfunction, and reduced cardiac output, all of which are exacerbated by dysregulated aldosterone.

Hypertension in Older Adults:

(hypertension) is one of the most common health issues faced by older adults, and aldosterone plays a key role in the development and progression of age-related hypertension. Aldosterone's sodium-retaining effects increase blood volume and vascular resistance, which contribute to elevated blood pressure. With aging, the

becomes less responsive to changes in blood volume and pressure, making it harder to regulate blood pressure effectively.

- **Mechanism of Action:** Aldosterone acts on the kidneys, where it promotes sodium reabsorption and water retention. This results in an increase in blood volume, which can raise blood pressure. In the elderly, the combined effects of **vascular stiffness, reduced kidney function**, and **impaired sodium handling** make it more difficult to regulate blood pressure despite aldosterone's action.
- **Clinical Implications:** Hypertension, if left unmanaged, can increase the risk of heart disease, stroke, kidney disease, and cognitive decline. Understanding the role of aldosterone in hypertension in older adults is crucial for effective treatment.

Heart Failure and Cardiac Remodeling:

cardiac remodeling

cardiac fibrosis

increased vascular resistance

myocardial stiffness

shortness of breath

fatigue

fluid retention

- **Aldosterone and Cardiac Remodeling:** The hormone promotes fibrosis in the heart tissue by stimulating the production of collagen and other extracellular matrix proteins. This process leads to thickening of the heart walls, which reduces its ability to contract and relax properly, contributing to heart failure.

- **Therapeutic Approaches:** Aldosterone antagonists like **spironolactone** and **eplerenone** are often used in the treatment of **heart failure** to block aldosterone's harmful effects on the heart. These medications have been shown to reduce mortality and improve symptoms in heart failure patients, especially those with **reduced ejection fraction**.

Vascular Stiffness and Endothelial Dysfunction:

endothelial dysfunction

Addressing Aldosterone Imbalance in Older Adults

Managing aldosterone imbalances in older adults is essential for preventing or mitigating the effects of hypertension, heart failure, and kidney disease. Several approaches can be taken to address these issues:

Aldosterone Antagonists:

spironolactone

eplerenone

heart failure

hypertension

chronic kidney disease

Benefits in Elderly Populations:

hyperkalemia

Lifestyle Modifications:

- **Dietary Modifications:** Reducing sodium intake, increasing potassium-rich foods, and maintaining adequate hydration can help balance aldosterone's effects on the kidneys and cardiovascular system.

- **Regular Exercise:** Physical activity is crucial for improving cardiovascular health, reducing blood pressure, and increasing the sensitivity of aldosterone receptors. Exercise can also help prevent and manage conditions like **diabetes**, which is commonly seen in the elderly and can exacerbate aldosterone imbalances.

- **Stress Management:** Chronic stress can increase aldosterone secretion, so adopting stress-reduction techniques such as mindfulness, meditation, and deep breathing exercises can help keep aldosterone levels in check.

3. **Monitoring Kidney Function:** Given the close relationship between aldosterone and kidney function, regular monitoring of kidney health is important, especially for older adults who may be at risk for **chronic kidney disease**. Monitoring **glomerular filtration rate (GFR)** and **serum creatinine** levels can help detect kidney dysfunction early and prevent further complications.

4. **Addressing Co-existing Conditions:** Many older adults with aldosterone imbalances have co-existing conditions such as **diabetes**, **obesity**, and **hyperlipidemia**. Managing these conditions through proper medication, diet, and exercise can help improve overall health and reduce the strain on aldosterone regulation.

Conclusion

Aging can significantly impact aldosterone secretion and its effects on the cardiovascular and renal systems. The combination of reduced renal function, changes in vascular stiffness, and the hormonal imbalances that accompany aging can exacerbate the adverse effects of aldosterone, contributing to hypertension, heart failure, and kidney disease. By addressing aldosterone imbalances through medications, lifestyle changes, and proper management of co-existing conditions, older adults can improve their overall health and mitigate the risks associated with aldosterone dysregulation. Understanding and mastering aldosterone in the context of aging will be crucial for enhancing the quality of life and longevity for the aging population.

Chapter 17: Targeting Aldosterone in the Treatment of Hypertension

Hypertension, or high blood pressure, is a widespread health issue that affects millions of people worldwide, with significant implications for cardiovascular and kidney health. One of the key factors in the development and persistence of hypertension is an imbalance in the **renin-angiotensin-aldosterone system (RAAS)**, which regulates fluid and sodium balance in the body. Aldosterone, a hormone produced by the adrenal glands, plays a central role in this system, and its dysregulation can contribute to sustained high blood pressure. In this chapter, we will explore the role of aldosterone in hypertension, the current treatments targeting aldosterone in managing high blood pressure, and the potential future of aldosterone-based therapies.

The Role of Aldosterone in Hypertension

Aldosterone contributes to hypertension primarily through its effects on **sodium retention**, **water retention**, and **vascular tone**. When aldosterone levels are elevated, it stimulates the kidneys to reabsorb sodium from urine, leading to increased water retention and an increase in blood volume. This elevated blood volume raises blood pressure. In addition to its renal effects, aldosterone has direct effects on the **blood vessels**, promoting vasoconstriction (narrowing of blood vessels), which further contributes to increased blood pressure.

Aldosterone's role in **secondary hypertension**—hypertension caused by another underlying health condition—is particularly significant. Conditions such as **primary aldosteronism, heart failure, chronic kidney disease**, and **renal artery stenosis** can cause an overproduction of aldosterone, exacerbating hypertension. In **primary aldosteronism**, the adrenal glands produce too much aldosterone independently of the normal regulatory mechanisms, leading to increased sodium retention and high blood pressure.

Thus, targeting aldosterone has become a key strategy in treating resistant hypertension, a form of high blood pressure that does not respond to standard treatments.

Treatment of Hypertension Involving Aldosterone Antagonists

Aldosterone antagonists, also known as **mineralocorticoid receptor antagonists (MRAs)**, are a class of drugs that block the effects of aldosterone on its receptor sites, thereby reducing its harmful effects on sodium and fluid retention, blood pressure, and cardiovascular function. Two main MRAs are commonly used in the treatment of hypertension:

Spironolactone:

- **Mechanism of Action:** By blocking aldosterone's effect on the kidneys, spironolactone helps prevent sodium retention and water accumulation, promoting **natriuresis** (the excretion of sodium in the urine). This reduces blood volume and helps lower blood pressure. In addition, spironolactone's ability to block aldosterone also prevents the **cardiac fibrosis** and **vascular remodeling** that are often seen in chronic hypertension.

- **Clinical Use:** Spironolactone is particularly effective in managing **resistant hypertension** (high blood pressure that does not respond to typical medications) and is used as a second- or third-line treatment in patients with **primary aldosteronism, heart failure**, or **chronic kidney disease**. It has also been found to improve **survival rates** and reduce **hospitalizations** in patients with **heart failure with reduced ejection fraction (HFrEF)**.

- **Side Effects:** While effective, spironolactone is not without side effects. It can cause **hyperkalemia** (elevated potassium levels), **gynecomastia** (enlargement of breast tissue in men), and **sexual dysfunction**. Monitoring potassium levels is essential during treatment to avoid complications from excessive potassium buildup.

Eplerenone:

- **Mechanism of Action:** Eplerenone selectively blocks the mineralocorticoid receptor, inhibiting aldosterone's effects on sodium retention, blood volume, and vascular tone. Its action in the kidneys helps lower blood pressure and reduce **cardiac fibrosis**.

- **Clinical Use:** Eplerenone is used in the treatment of hypertension, particularly in patients who cannot tolerate spironolactone due to side effects. It is also effective in patients with **heart failure** and **chronic kidney disease**. Like spironolactone, eplerenone is used in cases of **resistant hypertension** or when other antihypertensive medications are insufficient.

- **Side Effects:** Eplerenone is generally well-tolerated, but like spironolactone, it can lead to **hyperkalemia**, especially in patients with kidney impairment. Close monitoring of potassium and kidney function is required during treatment.

Combination Therapy:

combination therapy

ACE inhibitors

angiotensin II receptor blockers (ARBs)

calcium channel blockers

diuretics

Aldosterone-Based Hypertension Treatment: Benefits and Challenges

The use of aldosterone antagonists in the treatment of hypertension has significant benefits, particularly for individuals with **primary aldosteronism** or **heart failure**. However, the treatment comes with its own set of challenges that must be carefully managed:

1. **Hyperkalemia Risk:** Aldosterone antagonists can raise potassium levels, leading to **hyperkalemia** (high potassium levels). This can be dangerous if left unmonitored, especially in patients with kidney impairment or those taking other medications that affect potassium levels. Regular monitoring of **serum potassium** and **renal function** is essential to prevent complications from hyperkalemia.

2. **Kidney Function:** Both spironolactone and eplerenone can affect kidney function, particularly in patients with pre-existing kidney disease. In these cases, close monitoring of **glomerular filtration rate (GFR)** and **serum creatinine** levels is necessary to ensure kidney health is maintained during treatment.

3. **Individualized Treatment Plans:** As with any hypertension treatment, it is essential to tailor therapy to each individual. In the case of aldosterone antagonists, this means assessing the patient's overall health, kidney function, potassium levels, and any other comorbid conditions that might affect drug safety and efficacy.

4. **Adherence to Therapy:** Adherence to treatment regimens is crucial, especially in patients with **resistant hypertension**. Monitoring for side effects and educating patients on the importance of regular check-ups can help improve adherence and outcomes.

The Future of Aldosterone–Based Hypertension Treatments

The future of hypertension treatment is likely to involve more precise targeting of aldosterone and the RAAS system. As research advances, several exciting developments are emerging:

1. **Selective Mineralocorticoid Receptor Antagonists (MRAs):** Newer, more selective MRAs are being developed that may offer better outcomes with fewer side effects. For example, drugs that more specifically target aldosterone's actions on the heart and kidneys, while avoiding undesirable effects on other tissues, could revolutionize treatment.

2. **Gene Therapy and Molecular Approaches:** Emerging gene therapies may offer the potential to correct underlying genetic mutations or receptor sensitivities involved in aldosterone-related hypertension. This could lead to more permanent solutions rather than ongoing medication use.

3. **Combination Therapies with New Mechanisms:** The combination of MRAs with emerging drug classes that target different aspects of the RAAS or other pathways may offer enhanced efficacy in treating resistant hypertension. Ongoing research into combination therapies and their synergistic effects will likely improve treatment options for patients who do not respond to standard regimens.

Conclusion

Targeting aldosterone in the treatment of hypertension has proven to be an effective strategy, particularly in patients with **primary aldosteronism**, **heart failure**, and **chronic kidney disease**. Aldosterone antagonists, such as spironolactone and eplerenone, play a vital role in lowering blood pressure, improving heart failure outcomes, and preventing kidney damage. However, managing side effects like hyperkalemia and kidney dysfunction requires careful monitoring. As research advances, the development of more selective aldosterone-targeted therapies holds promise for improving hypertension management and enhancing patient outcomes. By understanding the critical role aldosterone plays in hypertension, healthcare providers can better address the complexities of managing high blood pressure, ultimately improving the health and quality of life for their patients.

Chapter 18: Natural Supplements and Herbs for Aldosterone Balance

Aldosterone is a key hormone involved in fluid balance, blood pressure regulation, and electrolyte homeostasis. When aldosterone is out of balance, it can lead to a variety of health conditions, including hypertension, heart disease, and kidney dysfunction. While pharmacological treatments such as aldosterone antagonists (spironolactone and eplerenone) are commonly prescribed to regulate aldosterone levels, natural supplements and herbs may offer additional support to help maintain aldosterone balance in the body. This chapter explores some of the most promising natural supplements and herbs that can help regulate aldosterone levels, improve fluid balance, and support overall health.

1. Magnesium: The Mineral that Modulates Aldosterone

Magnesium is a critical mineral that plays a role in numerous physiological processes, including **muscle function**, **nerve conduction**, and **electrolyte balance**. It also influences aldosterone secretion. Adequate magnesium levels have been shown to reduce aldosterone secretion, which can help prevent conditions such as **hypertension** and **fluid retention**.

- **Magnesium and Aldosterone Regulation:** Magnesium acts as a natural antagonist to calcium and sodium, which helps prevent the excessive action of aldosterone in the kidneys and other tissues. Magnesium is thought to block the sodium channels that aldosterone activates, thereby reducing the amount of sodium reabsorbed by the kidneys and preventing water retention.

- **Sources and Dosage:** Foods rich in magnesium, such as **leafy green vegetables, nuts, seeds**, and **whole grains**, can help maintain magnesium levels. In some cases, magnesium supplements may be recommended, especially for individuals who are magnesium-deficient or suffering from conditions related to aldosterone imbalance. Typical doses for magnesium supplementation range from **200-400 mg** per day, depending on individual needs.

2. Potassium: A Key Ally in Sodium and Aldosterone Balance

Potassium plays a crucial role in counterbalancing the effects of aldosterone by promoting sodium excretion. It helps prevent the negative effects of sodium retention, including high blood pressure and fluid buildup.

- **Potassium's Role in Aldosterone Balance:** High potassium intake can help lower aldosterone levels by reducing the need for aldosterone to retain sodium. Additionally, potassium helps to maintain proper heart function and normal blood pressure. This mineral is especially important in people taking aldosterone antagonists or those who experience **hypokalemia** (low potassium) due to excess aldosterone production.

- **Sources and Dosage:** A diet high in potassium-rich foods such as **bananas**, **oranges**, **sweet potatoes**, **spinach**, and **avocados** can support aldosterone balance. Potassium supplementation should be approached cautiously, as excessive intake can lead to **hyperkalemia** (high potassium levels). The recommended daily intake for potassium is approximately **2,500 to 3,000 mg** for most adults, but individual requirements may vary.

3. Coenzyme Q10 (CoQ10): A Powerful Antioxidant for Cardiovascular Health

Coenzyme Q10, also known as **ubiquinone**, is a naturally occurring antioxidant that plays a crucial role in cellular energy production and heart health. Research has shown that CoQ10 may help regulate aldosterone secretion and protect against cardiovascular complications caused by aldosterone dysregulation.

- **CoQ10 and Aldosterone Regulation:** CoQ10 can help improve endothelial function, reduce oxidative stress, and regulate blood pressure. Studies have suggested that CoQ10 supplementation may reduce aldosterone-induced damage to blood vessels and reduce the symptoms of **hypertension** and **heart failure**.

- **Sources and Dosage:** CoQ10 can be obtained through dietary sources such as **fatty fish, spinach, broccoli**, and **whole grains**, though the amounts from food sources may be insufficient for therapeutic effects. Supplementation is commonly used to support cardiovascular health, with doses ranging from **100-200 mg per day**.

4. Rhodiola Rosea: An Adaptogen for Stress Reduction

Rhodiola rosea is an **adaptogenic herb** that helps the body adapt to stress by balancing hormone levels and enhancing resilience to physical and mental stressors. This herb may also influence aldosterone secretion by modulating the **HPA axis** and reducing the effects of chronic stress on aldosterone production.

- **Rhodiola and Stress-Induced Aldosterone Secretion:** By lowering the production of **cortisol**, Rhodiola may help mitigate the activation of the **renin-angiotensin-aldosterone system (RAAS)** during periods of stress. This action can help prevent the increase in aldosterone levels that contributes to hypertension and fluid retention during stressful times.
- **Sources and Dosage:** Rhodiola rosea supplements are available in various forms, including capsules, tablets, and tinctures. The typical dosage is **200-400 mg** per day, though individuals may need to adjust based on their response and health needs.

5. Licorice Root: A Natural Diuretic

Licorice root has been used for centuries in traditional medicine for its anti-inflammatory and **diuretic properties**. However, licorice also has the potential to influence aldosterone levels by inhibiting the enzyme **11β-hydroxysteroid dehydrogenase type 2 (11β-HSD2)**, which normally converts **cortisol** to its inactive form, **cortisone**.

- **Licorice and Aldosterone:** When licorice inhibits 11β-HSD2, it may increase the effective concentration of cortisol, which can bind to mineralocorticoid receptors and mimic the effects of aldosterone, leading to sodium retention and increased blood pressure. While licorice has therapeutic benefits, excessive consumption can lead to **high blood pressure** and **low potassium** due to its aldosterone-like effects.

- **Sources and Dosage:** Licorice root can be consumed in the form of **teas**, **extracts**, or **tablets**. However, licorice should be used cautiously, and long-term use should be avoided, especially in individuals with **hypertension** or **kidney disease**. A typical dose ranges from **1-2 grams** per day, but this should be closely monitored to avoid side effects.

6. Ashwagandha: An Adaptogen for Adrenal Support

Ashwagandha is another **adaptogenic herb** that helps regulate the body's stress response by balancing cortisol levels. By reducing cortisol, ashwagandha may indirectly help reduce aldosterone secretion, since both hormones are closely linked through the **HPA axis**.

- **Ashwagandha and Aldosterone:** While research specifically linking ashwagandha to aldosterone regulation is limited, its role in reducing stress and balancing the HPA axis may have a positive impact on aldosterone secretion, particularly in individuals experiencing stress-related hypertension.

- **Sources and Dosage:** Ashwagandha is available in supplement form, typically in **capsules**, **powder**, or **extracts**. The recommended dosage is typically **300-600 mg** of standardized extract per day, although this may vary depending on individual health needs.

7. Omega–3 Fatty Acids: Reducing Inflammation and Supporting Heart Health

Omega-3 fatty acids, found in **fish oil** and **flaxseed**, are essential fats that support heart health and reduce inflammation. Omega-3s have been shown to have beneficial effects on **blood pressure, vascular health,** and **kidney function**, all of which are impacted by aldosterone.

- **Omega-3s and Aldosterone:** Omega-3 fatty acids may help reduce the harmful effects of high aldosterone, such as **vascular remodeling** and **fibrosis**. By supporting heart and kidney function and reducing systemic inflammation, omega-3s help mitigate the damaging effects of aldosterone dysregulation.

- **Sources and Dosage:** The best sources of omega-3s are **fatty fish** (salmon, mackerel, sardines) and **flaxseeds**. Omega-3 supplements, such as **fish oil** or **algal oil**, can be taken to achieve therapeutic levels, with a typical dose ranging from **1-3 grams** of EPA and DHA per day.

Conclusion

While pharmacological treatments such as **aldosterone antagonists** play a central role in managing aldosterone imbalances, natural supplements and herbs can provide complementary support in regulating aldosterone levels and improving overall health. Magnesium, potassium, CoQ10, Rhodiola, licorice root, ashwagandha, and omega-3 fatty acids are just a few of the natural agents that may help optimize aldosterone balance and support cardiovascular, renal, and metabolic health. As always, it is essential to consult with a healthcare professional before starting any new supplement regimen, particularly if you have underlying health conditions or are taking medications. By integrating these natural solutions into a holistic health approach, individuals can better manage aldosterone-related conditions and achieve long-term well-being.

Chapter 19: Advances in Aldosterone–Targeted Therapy

Aldosterone plays a critical role in the regulation of blood pressure, electrolyte balance, and fluid homeostasis. When it becomes dysregulated, it can lead to serious health conditions, including **hypertension, heart failure, chronic kidney disease**, and **electrolyte imbalances**. While traditional treatments like **aldosterone antagonists** (spironolactone and eplerenone) are commonly used, new advances in aldosterone-targeted therapies are offering promising opportunities for more precise, effective, and personalized treatments. This chapter explores the cutting-edge developments in aldosterone-targeted therapy, the role of aldosterone in new drug development, and what the future holds for aldosterone-based medicine.

1. Targeting the Aldosterone Receptor

The most common approach to managing aldosterone imbalance has been through **mineralocorticoid receptor antagonists (MRAs)**, such as spironolactone and eplerenone. These medications block aldosterone's effects at the **mineralocorticoid receptor**, primarily in the kidneys, heart, and blood vessels, which helps reduce sodium retention, water retention, and high blood pressure. However, while effective, these drugs have limitations, including side effects like **hyperkalemia** and **gynecomastia** (in the case of spironolactone).

- **Selective MRAs**: New research into more selective MRAs is providing therapies with fewer side effects and better targeting of aldosterone's effects. For example, **finerenone** is a novel selective mineralocorticoid receptor antagonist that has shown promise in clinical trials. Unlike spironolactone, finerenone has fewer adverse effects on potassium levels, making it a safer option for long-term use, particularly in patients with **chronic kidney disease** or **diabetes**.

- **Next-Generation MRAs**: These drugs focus on selectively blocking aldosterone without affecting other receptors in the body, such as the androgen receptor, which can cause side effects like gynecomastia. As these selective MRAs continue to improve, they may offer better tolerability and broader use in patients with cardiovascular and renal diseases.

2. Targeting the Renin–Angiotensin–Aldosterone System (RAAS)

The **RAAS** plays a central role in regulating aldosterone levels. In patients with hypertension or heart failure, the RAAS can become overactive, leading to increased aldosterone secretion. Current therapies that target RAAS include **ACE inhibitors** (angiotensin-converting enzyme inhibitors), **ARBs** (angiotensin receptor blockers), and **direct renin inhibitors**. These therapies can reduce aldosterone secretion indirectly by inhibiting the pathways that activate its release.

- **Dual RAAS Inhibition**: Recent studies have explored the benefits of combining **ACE inhibitors** or **ARBs** with aldosterone antagonists in a process known as dual RAAS inhibition. This approach has shown efficacy in controlling blood pressure and improving outcomes in conditions like **heart failure with reduced ejection fraction (HFrEF)**. However, the combination therapy is associated with an increased risk of hyperkalemia and kidney dysfunction, requiring close monitoring.

- **Direct Renin Inhibitors**: Another avenue of RAAS inhibition is through **direct renin inhibitors**, such as **aliskiren**. By targeting the enzyme renin, which is the first step in the RAAS cascade, these drugs prevent the production of angiotensin II and aldosterone. While effective in some patients, their use is limited due to potential adverse effects, including kidney dysfunction and hyperkalemia.

- **Gene Editing for RAAS**: One of the most exciting advances in RAAS-targeted therapies involves gene editing. By using techniques like **CRISPR-Cas9**, researchers are exploring the possibility of directly modifying the genes that control the production of angiotensin and aldosterone, potentially offering a more permanent solution to RAAS dysregulation.

3. Combining Therapies for Resistant Hypertension

Resistant hypertension, defined as blood pressure that remains elevated despite the use of three or more antihypertensive medications, is a growing concern in the medical community. Aldosterone dysregulation is a common factor in this condition. Combination therapies that include aldosterone antagonists alongside other blood pressure medications are showing promise in improving outcomes for these patients.

- **Aldosterone Antagonists with Calcium Channel Blockers**: Combining MRAs with **calcium channel blockers** (CCBs) can enhance blood pressure control by targeting different mechanisms in the vascular system. CCBs relax blood vessels and reduce vascular resistance, while MRAs counteract aldosterone-induced sodium and fluid retention. This combination has been shown to be particularly effective in managing resistant hypertension.

- **Aldosterone Antagonists and Diuretics**: Another combination strategy is pairing aldosterone antagonists with **thiazide diuretics** or **loop diuretics**. Diuretics help the body eliminate excess sodium and water, which complements the sodium-reducing effects of MRAs. This combination approach is frequently used in the management of **heart failure** and **chronic kidney disease**.

- **Fixed-Dose Combinations**: To improve patient adherence and reduce pill burden, researchers are developing fixed-dose combination therapies that include an aldosterone antagonist, a calcium channel blocker, and/or a diuretic. These combinations may help ensure better patient compliance, particularly in the elderly population, where polypharmacy is common.

4. Targeting Aldosterone Synthesis

Another exciting direction in aldosterone-targeted therapy is inhibiting the **synthesis of aldosterone** directly. Drugs that inhibit the enzymes responsible for aldosterone synthesis, particularly **11β-hydroxylase** and **aldosterone synthase (CYP11B2)**, are being investigated. These enzymes are responsible for the final steps in aldosterone production, and targeting them could provide a novel strategy for controlling aldosterone levels.

- **CYP11B2 Inhibitors**: Inhibition of the aldosterone synthase enzyme, which is responsible for the final step in aldosterone synthesis, offers the potential to reduce aldosterone levels in a more direct way. This approach could provide an effective solution for conditions like **primary aldosteronism** and **resistant hypertension**, where aldosterone plays a major role in disease progression.
- **Steroidogenesis Inhibitors**: **Steroidogenesis inhibitors**, such as **abiraterone**, which block enzymes involved in steroid hormone production, are being explored for their potential to reduce aldosterone secretion in certain conditions. These drugs are primarily used in the treatment of prostate cancer but could have broader applications in aldosterone-driven diseases.

5. Advances in Personalized Medicine

The future of aldosterone-based therapy is increasingly moving toward **personalized medicine**, which tailors treatment to individual patients based on their genetic makeup, underlying health conditions, and specific hormone profiles. Advances in **genetic testing** and **biomarker discovery** are paving the way for more targeted and effective treatments for aldosterone-related disorders.

- **Genetic Profiling**: By identifying genetic variations that affect aldosterone synthesis and receptor activity, healthcare providers can predict which patients are at higher risk for aldosterone imbalances and adjust their treatments accordingly. This could lead to more precise dosing and better management of conditions like **primary aldosteronism** and **resistant hypertension**.

- **Biomarkers for Monitoring Treatment**: The development of biomarkers to monitor aldosterone levels and the effectiveness of treatment is another promising area of research. By using biomarkers such as **plasma renin activity** or **aldosterone-to-renin ratio**, clinicians can better assess the effectiveness of aldosterone-targeted therapies and adjust treatment plans in real-time.

Conclusion

Advances in aldosterone-targeted therapies are changing the way we manage aldosterone dysregulation in conditions such as hypertension, heart failure, and chronic kidney disease. From more selective mineralocorticoid receptor antagonists to genetic and enzyme-targeting strategies, the future of aldosterone-based treatment holds great promise for improving outcomes and reducing the burden of cardiovascular and renal diseases. As research continues to uncover new ways to target aldosterone more precisely, personalized and combination therapies will likely play a central role in achieving optimal health and well-being for patients with aldosterone-related disorders. Through these innovations, we are on the cusp of a new era in the treatment of aldosterone imbalance, offering patients better, more effective therapies and a brighter future for managing hormone-related diseases.

Chapter 20: Conclusion: Mastering Aldosterone for Optimal Health

Aldosterone is far more than just a hormone that regulates fluid balance and blood pressure. Its influence extends throughout the body, touching on everything from **heart health** to **renal function** and even **brain activity**. As we have explored throughout this book, aldosterone plays a pivotal role in maintaining electrolyte balance and fluid volume, both of which are critical for health. When its regulation goes awry, it can lead to a variety of chronic conditions, including **hypertension, heart failure, kidney disease**, and **stroke risk**. However, mastering aldosterone—through a combination of targeted therapies, lifestyle changes, and natural remedies—holds the key to preventing and managing these conditions.

1. Understanding Aldosterone's Role in Health

Aldosterone's primary function is to regulate sodium and potassium levels through its action on the kidneys. By increasing sodium reabsorption and potassium excretion, aldosterone helps maintain blood volume and blood pressure. However, excessive or insufficient production of aldosterone can have detrimental effects on the body, leading to **fluid retention, elevated blood pressure**, and **electrolyte imbalances**. Furthermore, aldosterone's action is interconnected with other critical hormones and systems, such as **cortisol** (through the **HPA axis**) and **angiotensin II** (through the **RAAS system**), making its regulation an intricate and essential component of overall hormonal balance.

2. Addressing Aldosterone Imbalance

As we've learned in previous chapters, aldosterone imbalances can result in various conditions:

- **Primary Aldosteronism (Conn's Syndrome)**: Overproduction of aldosterone due to adrenal gland tumors or hyperplasia can lead to high blood pressure, potassium deficiency, and increased risk for stroke or heart disease.
- **Secondary Hyperaldosteronism**: This occurs when aldosterone is elevated due to excessive renin production, often seen in conditions like **heart failure, liver cirrhosis**, and **renal artery stenosis**.
- **Addison's Disease**: Insufficient aldosterone secretion in **Addison's disease** leads to **electrolyte imbalances, fatigue**, and **low blood pressure**.

Each of these conditions requires a tailored approach to treatment, involving a combination of pharmacological interventions (like aldosterone antagonists), lifestyle changes (including sodium and fluid regulation), and in some cases, surgical procedures. Understanding the root cause of aldosterone dysregulation is essential for choosing the right course of treatment.

3. The Future of Aldosterone Management: Advancing Therapy and Personalization

As the understanding of aldosterone's role in health expands, new treatments are emerging to more effectively manage its dysregulation. The future of aldosterone-targeted therapies holds great promise, particularly with advancements in **genetic profiling, precision medicine**, and **novel drug development**. Here are a few of the key developments on the horizon:

- **Gene Editing**: Advances in **CRISPR-Cas9** technology may one day enable precise genetic interventions to alter aldosterone production at the DNA level, potentially offering a long-term solution for patients with inherited conditions like **primary aldosteronism**.

- **Targeted Mineralocorticoid Receptor Antagonists**: As we've discussed, **finerenone** is a more selective MRA that offers a safer profile for patients with **chronic kidney disease** or **diabetes**. Continued research into MRAs may lead to even more refined therapies with fewer side effects.

- **Biomarkers for Aldosterone Imbalance**: The development of specific biomarkers for aldosterone-related diseases will enhance early diagnosis and allow for more effective monitoring of treatment efficacy. This will help guide therapy, making treatment more personalized and precise.

- **Combination Therapies**: The combination of aldosterone-targeting drugs with other antihypertensive medications, like **calcium channel blockers** or **angiotensin receptor blockers (ARBs)**, may offer enhanced control of blood pressure in patients with resistant hypertension, allowing for better outcomes and fewer side effects.

4. The Role of Lifestyle in Mastering Aldosterone

While medications and advanced therapies play a significant role in managing aldosterone imbalances, lifestyle changes are just as important. Proper **hydration**, a balanced **diet**, regular **exercise**, and **stress management** can have a profound impact on aldosterone levels and the body's ability to maintain fluid and electrolyte balance.

- **Hydration**: Proper fluid intake is crucial for balancing sodium and aldosterone. Dehydration can trigger aldosterone release to conserve sodium, while overhydration can reduce aldosterone secretion. Ensuring adequate water intake and avoiding excessive salt or sugar intake can help maintain aldosterone regulation.

- **Diet**: A balanced diet rich in potassium and magnesium (which help mitigate the effects of excess aldosterone) and low in sodium can support aldosterone balance. The Mediterranean diet, which emphasizes whole foods, healthy fats, fruits, and vegetables, is particularly beneficial.

- **Exercise**: Regular exercise helps maintain healthy blood pressure and reduces the stress that can elevate aldosterone levels. Moderate physical activity supports cardiovascular health, improves kidney function, and helps with weight management—key factors in managing aldosterone levels.

- **Stress Reduction**: Chronic stress activates the **HPA axis**, leading to the release of cortisol and stimulating aldosterone secretion. Practices such as **mindfulness, yoga**, and **meditation** can help reduce stress and support hormonal balance.

5. Key Takeaways for Mastering Aldosterone

To master aldosterone and its effects on your health, consider the following actionable strategies:

- **Regular Monitoring**: Keep track of your blood pressure, electrolyte levels, and kidney function with the help of your healthcare provider. Regular testing of aldosterone, renin, and other related markers can help catch any imbalances early.

- **Balanced Nutrition**: Focus on a nutrient-rich diet that supports aldosterone balance, including foods high in **potassium** and **magnesium** while limiting sodium intake.

- **Personalized Treatment**: Work closely with your healthcare provider to identify the best treatment plan, whether it involves **aldosterone antagonists**, **RAAS inhibitors**, or newer therapies. Genetic testing may help tailor treatments for more effective management of aldosterone-related conditions.

- **Holistic Health**: Adopt a holistic approach that incorporates **stress management**, **exercise**, and **adequate hydration** to optimize your body's ability to maintain fluid and electrolyte balance.

6. Final Thoughts on Maintaining Hormonal Balance for Longevity and Vitality

Mastering aldosterone is essential for maintaining fluid balance, blood pressure regulation, and overall health. By understanding its intricate role in the body and addressing imbalances with targeted therapies, lifestyle modifications, and natural remedies, you can prevent and manage aldosterone-related disorders.

As science continues to advance in aldosterone-targeted therapies and personalized medicine, the future holds great promise for more effective treatments and better patient outcomes. With careful attention to **diet, exercise, stress management**, and **medical treatment**, you can master aldosterone and pave the way for a long, healthy life with optimal hormonal balance.

Chapter 21: Key Takeaways and Actionable Strategies

In this final chapter, we summarize the most important insights from our exploration of aldosterone, its role in the body, and the strategies for managing its balance. Understanding aldosterone and how it influences fluid balance, blood pressure regulation, and overall hormonal health is crucial for maintaining optimal health. Whether you are dealing with aldosterone-related conditions or simply seeking to optimize your well-being, mastering aldosterone is key to preventing and managing a variety of health concerns.

1. Understanding Aldosterone's Role in the Body

Aldosterone is a steroid hormone produced by the adrenal glands that regulates sodium and potassium levels in the body, directly influencing blood volume and pressure. Its effects are essential for maintaining fluid balance, electrolyte regulation, and proper kidney function. Disruption in aldosterone levels can lead to a range of conditions, from **hypertension** and **heart failure** to **kidney disease** and **stroke**.

- **Excessive aldosterone** leads to fluid retention, sodium imbalance, and elevated blood pressure.

- **Insufficient aldosterone** causes electrolyte imbalances, dehydration, and low blood pressure.

- Proper management of aldosterone is vital for maintaining cardiovascular and renal health.

2. Managing Aldosterone Imbalances

Aldosterone dysregulation can result in conditions like **primary aldosteronism**, **secondary hyperaldosteronism**, and **Addison's disease**, each requiring tailored treatment strategies:

- **Primary Aldosteronism (Conn's Syndrome)**: Overproduction of aldosterone due to adrenal tumors or hyperplasia can cause hypertension and potassium deficiency. Treatment options include surgical removal of the tumor or medical management with **aldosterone antagonists** (e.g., spironolactone, eplerenone).

- **Secondary Hyperaldosteronism**: Caused by conditions such as heart failure or renal artery stenosis, this results in excessive renin secretion and aldosterone production. Treatment focuses on addressing the underlying cause and managing blood pressure with RAAS inhibitors.

- **Addison's Disease**: Characterized by insufficient aldosterone, leading to low blood pressure and electrolyte imbalances. Treatment typically involves **mineralocorticoid replacement therapy**, such as fludrocortisone, to normalize aldosterone levels.

3. Pharmacological Approaches to Target Aldosterone

Pharmacological treatments play a central role in managing aldosterone-related disorders. The most common approaches include:

- **Aldosterone Antagonists**: These drugs, such as **spironolactone** and **eplerenone**, block aldosterone's action at the mineralocorticoid receptor in the kidneys, heart, and blood vessels. They are used in conditions like **hypertension, heart failure**, and **chronic kidney disease**. Side effects, such as **hyperkalemia** and **gynecomastia** (inspironolactone), are common, but newer agents like **finerenone** offer better safety profiles.

- **RAAS Inhibitors**: ACE inhibitors, angiotensin receptor blockers (ARBs), and **direct renin inhibitors** reduce aldosterone production by targeting the RAAS. These are often combined with aldosterone antagonists to manage **resistant hypertension** and **heart failure**.

- **Steroidogenesis Inhibitors**: Emerging treatments involve inhibiting aldosterone synthesis via **aldosterone synthase inhibitors** or **11β-hydroxylase inhibitors**, which could offer a novel approach for treating aldosterone-related conditions.

4. Lifestyle Modifications for Optimizing Aldosterone Function

While medications are essential for managing aldosterone dysregulation, **lifestyle modifications** are equally important in maintaining balance and optimizing aldosterone function. Consider these actionable strategies:

- **Hydration**: Ensure adequate fluid intake to avoid dehydration, which can trigger aldosterone release. However, avoid excessive water retention by regulating sodium intake. Maintaining optimal hydration helps to balance aldosterone and prevent its overproduction or underproduction.

- **Dietary Adjustments**: A diet rich in **potassium** (e.g., bananas, leafy greens, and potatoes) and **magnesium** (e.g., nuts, seeds, and whole grains) helps offset the effects of excess aldosterone. Reducing **sodium** intake is crucial for managing high aldosterone levels, while increasing **fiber** intake can promote overall cardiovascular health.

- **Regular Exercise**: Exercise helps to regulate blood pressure and reduce aldosterone production by enhancing blood flow and improving cardiovascular health. Aim for moderate physical activity, such as walking, swimming, or cycling, to help balance aldosterone levels and support overall heart health.

- **Stress Reduction**: Chronic stress activates the **HPA axis**, increasing cortisol levels and stimulating aldosterone release. Managing stress through techniques like **meditation, yoga**, and **deep breathing** can help keep aldosterone and cortisol levels in check.

5. Integrative Approaches for Comprehensive Health

While conventional treatments are vital, **integrative approaches** incorporating traditional and alternative therapies can complement medical management of aldosterone imbalances. Consider these practices for a more holistic approach:

- **Natural Supplements**: Certain supplements may support aldosterone balance, including **omega-3 fatty acids** (anti-inflammatory), **magnesium** (for electrolyte balance), and **adaptogenic herbs** like **ashwagandha** (to reduce stress). Always consult a healthcare provider before incorporating supplements into your routine.

- **Herbal Remedies**: **Hibiscus tea**, **garlic**, and **parsley** are believed to have mild diuretic and blood pressure-lowering effects, potentially supporting aldosterone regulation. However, these should not replace prescribed medications but may serve as complementary treatments.

- **Traditional Medicine**: Practices such as **acupuncture** and **traditional Chinese medicine (TCM)** may help in managing stress and promoting overall health, indirectly supporting aldosterone balance.

6. Monitoring and Measuring Aldosterone Levels

Regular monitoring of aldosterone levels, as well as related biomarkers like **plasma renin activity** and **serum potassium levels**, is crucial for assessing treatment effectiveness and ensuring that aldosterone imbalances are appropriately managed. Blood and urine tests are commonly used to measure aldosterone levels, helping to identify the underlying causes of any imbalances and guide treatment decisions.

7. Key Takeaways for Mastering Aldosterone

- **Regular Monitoring**: Monitor blood pressure, electrolyte levels, and kidney function regularly to detect early signs of aldosterone imbalance.

- **Balanced Nutrition**: Focus on a potassium-rich, sodium-controlled diet that promotes aldosterone balance. The Mediterranean diet is an excellent model.

- **Pharmacological Management**: Work with healthcare providers to find the best treatment options, including aldosterone antagonists, RAAS inhibitors, or newer therapies, depending on individual needs.

- **Lifestyle Adjustments**: Implement stress management techniques, maintain hydration, and engage in regular physical activity to optimize aldosterone regulation.

- **Integrative Approaches**: Explore complementary treatments like supplements, herbs, and traditional medicine for added support in balancing aldosterone and improving overall health.

8. Final Thoughts on Maintaining Hormonal Balance for Longevity and Vitality

Mastering aldosterone is crucial for maintaining hormonal balance and optimizing long-term health. By understanding its role in fluid and blood pressure regulation and taking steps to address imbalances, you can reduce the risk of chronic diseases such as hypertension, heart failure, and kidney disease. With the right combination of medical treatment, lifestyle choices, and holistic health practices, you can unlock the secrets to balancing aldosterone, promoting well-being, and achieving longevity and vitality.

In conclusion, achieving optimal aldosterone balance requires a comprehensive, individualized approach that includes early detection, treatment, and lifestyle management. By mastering aldosterone, you take control of your health, paving the way for a future of vitality and resilience.

Chapter 22: Conclusion: Mastering Aldosterone for Optimal Health

Throughout this book, we've explored aldosterone's vital role in maintaining fluid balance, regulating blood pressure, and ensuring overall hormonal health. Aldosterone, a key hormone produced by the adrenal glands, influences several systems within the body, including the cardiovascular, renal, and neurovascular systems. Its impact on electrolyte regulation, blood pressure, and kidney function cannot be overstated.

Now, as we conclude our journey into mastering aldosterone, let's review the key takeaways and actionable strategies that can help you achieve better health outcomes through understanding and managing aldosterone balance.

1. The Central Role of Aldosterone in Fluid and Electrolyte Balance

Aldosterone is essential in regulating sodium and potassium levels, which in turn, influence water balance and blood pressure. It operates within the **Renin-Angiotensin-Aldosterone System (RAAS)**, a complex cascade that responds to changes in blood pressure, volume, and sodium levels.

- **Sodium retention** by the kidneys increases blood volume, which raises blood pressure.
- **Potassium excretion** is essential for maintaining proper electrolyte levels.
- Disruptions in aldosterone levels can lead to conditions such as **hypertension**, **hypokalemia**, and **heart failure**.

Mastering aldosterone requires a deep understanding of how these physiological processes work together to maintain equilibrium in the body.

2. Aldosterone Imbalances and Health Implications

When aldosterone levels are too high or too low, they can lead to serious health conditions:

- **Excess aldosterone** can lead to **primary aldosteronism**, resulting in high blood pressure, low potassium, and potential cardiovascular damage. Secondary hyperaldosteronism, often seen in **heart failure** and **kidney disease**, also involves elevated aldosterone levels as a response to underlying conditions.
- **Aldosterone deficiency**, as seen in **Addison's disease**, leads to low blood pressure, fatigue, and electrolyte imbalances.

Recognizing the symptoms of aldosterone imbalance and seeking appropriate medical attention is crucial. Early detection and intervention can significantly improve long-term health outcomes.

3. Pharmacological Approaches to Managing Aldosterone

Treatment options for aldosterone-related conditions primarily involve **RAAS inhibitors**, **aldosterone antagonists**, and sometimes **surgical interventions**.

- **Spironolactone** and **eplerenone** are commonly used to block aldosterone's action, particularly in treating **hypertension, heart failure**, and **kidney disease**. These medications help prevent fluid retention and lower blood pressure.
- **ACE inhibitors** and **ARBs** also inhibit aldosterone production, further supporting the management of blood pressure and heart function.

When using these pharmacological agents, it's important to monitor for side effects, such as **hyperkalemia** and **kidney dysfunction**, ensuring the treatments are tailored to the individual's health needs.

4. Lifestyle Strategies to Support Aldosterone Balance

While medications are important for managing aldosterone imbalances, lifestyle modifications can enhance the effectiveness of treatment and prevent complications. Here are key strategies for supporting aldosterone function:

- **Balanced Nutrition**: A diet high in **potassium** (e.g., bananas, leafy greens) and **magnesium** (e.g., nuts, seeds) and low in **sodium** can help balance aldosterone levels.

- **Hydration**: Proper hydration helps maintain aldosterone levels, as dehydration can trigger excessive aldosterone release. However, excessive water retention, caused by high sodium levels, can counteract aldosterone balance.

- **Exercise**: Regular physical activity promotes blood flow and supports healthy blood pressure levels, reducing the strain on the cardiovascular system and kidneys. Exercise also helps reduce stress, which can affect aldosterone secretion.

- **Stress Management**: Chronic stress can increase cortisol levels, which in turn may affect aldosterone secretion. Using techniques such as **meditation**, **yoga**, and **deep breathing** exercises can significantly improve aldosterone regulation.

5. Integrative Approaches for Comprehensive Health

Traditional and alternative therapies can complement conventional treatments in managing aldosterone imbalances. Consider the following integrative approaches:

- **Herbal Supplements**: Certain herbs, such as **garlic**, **hibiscus**, and **parsley**, are believed to have mild diuretic and blood pressure-lowering effects that could support aldosterone regulation.

- **Adaptogens**: Herbs like **ashwagandha** may help regulate the body's stress response, indirectly supporting aldosterone balance.

- **Acupuncture**: This traditional practice has been shown to help reduce stress and support overall health, potentially improving the body's ability to maintain aldosterone equilibrium.

Always consult a healthcare provider before introducing herbal supplements or alternative therapies, as they may interact with prescription medications.

6. Advancing Research and Treatment for Aldosterone Disorders

The future of aldosterone research holds exciting promise for advancing treatments and improving our understanding of aldosterone-related disorders:

- **Genetic Testing**: Understanding genetic mutations that influence aldosterone production can lead to personalized treatments for individuals with genetic predispositions to **hypertension** and **heart disease**.
- **New Drug Development**: Advances in aldosterone-targeted therapies, such as **aldosterone synthase inhibitors**, may offer new treatment options for resistant cases of hypertension and heart failure.
- **Precision Medicine**: The development of therapies tailored to a patient's unique genetic and physiological makeup could revolutionize the treatment of aldosterone-related conditions.

7. Monitoring and Long-Term Health Management

Ongoing monitoring of aldosterone levels is crucial for individuals at risk for aldosterone imbalances. Regular blood tests and urine samples, along with monitoring blood pressure and kidney function, will help detect imbalances early and ensure treatment efficacy.

- **Healthcare providers** should regularly assess aldosterone-related biomarkers and adapt treatment plans as necessary.
- **Self-monitoring** of blood pressure, weight, and electrolyte levels (such as potassium) can provide valuable insights into the effectiveness of the treatment regimen.

8. The Path Forward: Maintaining Hormonal Balance

Ultimately, **mastering aldosterone** is about maintaining hormonal balance to optimize long-term health. By recognizing the signs of aldosterone imbalances, understanding the physiological mechanisms at play, and implementing appropriate treatment strategies, you can enhance your overall well-being.

The combination of pharmacological treatments, lifestyle modifications, and integrative approaches will empower you to take control of your health and live a life marked by vitality, balance, and longevity.

In conclusion, mastering aldosterone is a journey toward **optimal health**, requiring both proactive management and ongoing awareness. By integrating the insights gained throughout this book, you can support your body's natural regulatory mechanisms and ensure a healthier future. Whether you're dealing with aldosterone-related disorders or simply optimizing your health, understanding and managing aldosterone is a crucial step on the path to well-being.

Final Thoughts: Hormonal balance, particularly with aldosterone, is at the core of our health. By actively working to maintain this balance through thoughtful strategies, you can unlock a future of health, vitality, and longevity.

Chapter 23: The Role of Aldosterone in New Drug Development: Paving the Way for Better Health

In this chapter, we will explore the cutting-edge research and developments in aldosterone-targeted therapies. As our understanding of aldosterone and its profound influence on health continues to grow, it is clear that the future of medical treatments will increasingly focus on optimizing aldosterone regulation. This includes novel drug interventions, innovative therapies, and the potential for personalized medicine that takes into account an individual's unique genetic makeup.

1. Current Aldosterone–Targeted Therapies

The most widely used drugs for managing aldosterone imbalances include **aldosterone antagonists** like **spironolactone** and **eplerenone**, which are commonly prescribed for conditions such as **hypertension, heart failure**, and **kidney disease**. These medications work by blocking the action of aldosterone at its receptor, preventing the hormone from inducing excessive sodium retention, which helps control blood pressure and fluid balance.

While these drugs have been effective in managing the symptoms of aldosterone imbalances, they come with limitations and side effects, such as **hyperkalemia** (high potassium levels), which can pose significant health risks. Spironolactone, for instance, has anti-androgenic effects, which may result in undesirable side effects like **gynecomastia** in men.

Despite these concerns, aldosterone antagonists represent a cornerstone in managing cardiovascular disease and renal failure. However, the need for more specific, targeted therapies with fewer side effects has driven the development of new approaches.

2. Advancements in Aldosterone-Targeted Therapies

Several promising new directions are being explored in the development of drugs that can better modulate aldosterone function without causing adverse side effects. These advancements include:

- **Aldosterone Synthase Inhibitors**: Researchers are working on developing drugs that inhibit the synthesis of aldosterone directly. By blocking **aldosterone synthase** (the enzyme responsible for aldosterone production), these drugs could reduce the hormone's secretion at its source, potentially offering a more direct and effective approach to controlling aldosterone levels. This type of drug could offer a more specific solution than current aldosterone antagonists.

- **Mineralocorticoid Receptor Blockers (MRBs)**: New classes of **mineralocorticoid receptor blockers** are under investigation. These drugs target the receptor more selectively and may be able to block aldosterone's effects without triggering the negative side effects that affect the kidneys and other organs. This specificity is a key advantage, as it reduces the risk of complications like electrolyte imbalances and kidney damage.

- **Combination Therapy**: The future of aldosterone treatment may also lie in combination therapies. For instance, combining **angiotensin-converting enzyme inhibitors (ACE inhibitors)** or **angiotensin receptor blockers (ARBs)** with selective aldosterone blockers could provide a synergistic effect in treating hypertension, heart failure, and kidney disease. By targeting multiple pathways in the RAAS, this approach may offer more comprehensive control over blood pressure and fluid

3. Personalized Medicine and Genetics
balance while minimizing side effects.

As we look to the future of aldosterone treatment, **personalized medicine** will play a crucial role. Genetic testing allows for a better understanding of individual variability in aldosterone metabolism, receptor sensitivity, and response to treatment. Researchers are beginning to uncover genetic mutations that impact aldosterone production and action, which will help in:

- **Tailoring Treatments**: Personalized approaches will ensure that individuals receive the most appropriate treatment based on their genetic profile. Some people may respond better to aldosterone antagonists, while others may benefit more from drugs that inhibit aldosterone synthesis or receptor blockers.

- **Predicting Drug Responses**: Genetic testing may also help predict how a patient will respond to certain drugs, minimizing trial and error in treatment and reducing the risk of adverse effects. This is especially important for managing chronic conditions like heart failure or kidney disease, where effective aldosterone control is critical for long-term outcomes.

4. Exploring the Intersection of Aldosterone and Other Hormones

Emerging research suggests that aldosterone does not function in isolation; rather, it interacts closely with other hormones and systems in the body. Understanding these interactions opens up new avenues for drug development:

- **Aldosterone and Cortisol**: The interplay between aldosterone and cortisol, the stress hormone, is of particular interest. Cortisol has been shown to influence aldosterone secretion, and drugs targeting both hormones could be more effective in treating conditions like **hypertension** and **stress-related disorders**.

- **Aldosterone and Sex Hormones**: The effects of aldosterone on sex hormones, particularly in **women**, are also gaining attention. Female sex hormones, such as **estrogen**, can influence aldosterone sensitivity and its effects on blood pressure regulation. Exploring how aldosterone interacts with these hormones could lead to more gender-specific treatments for aldosterone-related conditions.

5. Clinical Trials and the Path to Approval

As the science behind aldosterone-targeted therapies advances, the next step involves rigorous **clinical trials** to test the safety, efficacy, and long-term effects of these new treatments. Several promising compounds are currently undergoing clinical trials, with researchers focused on:

- Assessing **efficacy** in reducing aldosterone-related complications, such as hypertension and heart failure exacerbation.
- Monitoring **side effects**, including kidney function, electrolyte imbalances, and other potential toxicities.
- Exploring **long-term outcomes** for patients who are treated with these advanced therapies, ensuring they not only manage symptoms but also improve quality of life and reduce the risk of chronic conditions.

The regulatory approval process for these drugs is complex, requiring thorough data collection and analysis. However, as evidence accumulates, these therapies could become a central part of clinical practice for managing aldosterone imbalances.

6. The Future of Aldosterone–Based Medicine

The future of aldosterone-based medicine holds incredible promise. As we better understand the molecular mechanisms underlying aldosterone regulation and its role in health and disease, new therapies will emerge that are more precise, effective, and personalized than ever before.

Key innovations include:

- **Gene therapy**, which could potentially target the genes responsible for aldosterone production or receptor function.
- **MicroRNA-based therapies**, which could offer a way to regulate aldosterone at the genetic level, preventing overproduction of the hormone without affecting other systems in the body.

These advancements could revolutionize the way we approach aldosterone-related diseases, offering new hope to patients with heart disease, kidney failure, and other conditions linked to aldosterone dysregulation.

7. Conclusion: Shaping the Future of Aldosterone Health

Mastering aldosterone is not just about understanding its current role in human physiology; it is about unlocking new pathways for treatment and exploring the future of **personalized** and **precision medicine**. By advancing our knowledge of aldosterone and its interactions with other systems, we are on the cusp of a new era of targeted therapies that can dramatically improve health outcomes for individuals struggling with aldosterone imbalances.

As the future unfolds, we can expect to see more specific, effective treatments emerge, bringing better control over aldosterone's impact on blood pressure, heart health, and overall fluid balance. The potential for improving patient care and quality of life through aldosterone-targeted therapies is vast, and the ongoing research holds the key to unlocking optimal hormonal health for generations to come.

Chapter 24: Conclusion: Mastering Aldosterone for Optimal Health

As we have explored throughout this book, aldosterone is a key regulator of fluid balance, blood pressure, and overall hormonal health. From its intricate role in the **Renin-Angiotensin-Aldosterone System (RAAS)** to its significant impacts on the cardiovascular, renal, and neurovascular systems, aldosterone's influence on health is profound and far-reaching. Understanding and mastering aldosterone regulation is crucial not only for managing **hypertension**, **heart failure**, **kidney disease**, and a host of other conditions but also for promoting overall wellness and longevity.

In this final chapter, we will review the critical takeaways from the preceding sections, highlight actionable strategies for mastering aldosterone regulation in everyday life, and look toward future developments in aldosterone-related therapies.

Key Takeaways:

1. **Aldosterone's Essential Role in Fluid and Electrolyte Balance:** Aldosterone's primary function is to maintain **homeostasis** by regulating sodium and potassium balance. By promoting sodium reabsorption in the kidneys, it helps control blood volume and, consequently, blood pressure. Its intricate relationship with other hormones, particularly **cortisol** and **angiotensin II**, emphasizes its significance in overall physiological regulation.

2. **The Link Between Aldosterone and Hypertension:** Chronic elevation of aldosterone levels leads to **high blood pressure** (hypertension), a condition that can result in serious cardiovascular complications, including **stroke, heart attack,** and **renal failure.** Understanding the mechanisms by which aldosterone promotes sodium retention and blood pressure elevation is crucial in diagnosing and treating hypertension, especially in patients with **primary aldosteronism** (Conn's syndrome) and **secondary hyperaldosteronism.**

3. **Aldosterone and the Kidneys:** Aldosterone's interaction with the kidneys plays a vital role in regulating **renal function** and maintaining **fluid balance.** It is crucial for **sodium retention,** which is directly linked to blood pressure control, and for the regulation of **potassium** and **hydrogen ions.** Disruptions in aldosterone production can lead to electrolyte imbalances and kidney dysfunction, which are major concerns in **diabetic nephropathy** and **chronic kidney disease.**

4. **Aldosterone and Heart Health:** The hormone's impact on **cardiac remodeling** underscores its importance in managing **heart failure**. By increasing sodium retention, aldosterone promotes fluid accumulation, increasing the workload on the heart and exacerbating symptoms in patients with heart failure. Targeting aldosterone with **spironolactone** and **eplerenone** has shown significant benefits in improving patient outcomes and reducing mortality in heart failure treatment.

5. **Advances in Aldosterone-Based Therapies:** Research into more targeted **aldosterone blockers, aldosterone synthase inhibitors,** and **mineralocorticoid receptor antagonists (MRAs)** is promising, providing more specific and effective treatment options. These advancements aim to reduce side effects and improve patient outcomes, particularly in conditions such as **heart failure, hypertension,** and **chronic kidney disease**.

6. **Genetic and Hormonal Interactions:** The genetic basis of aldosterone regulation, including its interaction with **angiotensin II** and **cortisol**, is a critical area of research. Genetic testing is increasingly being used to predict responses to treatment and customize therapies for better management of aldosterone-related conditions. Future therapeutic approaches may include **gene therapy** or **microRNA interventions** to more precisely control aldosterone synthesis and action.

7. **The Impact of Diet and Lifestyle:** Diet and lifestyle choices significantly influence aldosterone regulation. Adequate **hydration**, maintaining a **balanced diet** low in sodium and rich in **potassium**, and engaging in regular **exercise** all play important roles in supporting healthy aldosterone levels. **Stress management** is another key factor, as chronic stress can trigger aldosterone release and exacerbate hypertension and other cardiovascular conditions.

Actionable Strategies for Mastering Aldosterone Regulation:

1. **Monitor and Manage Sodium Intake:** Reducing sodium consumption is one of the most effective ways to maintain healthy aldosterone levels. Excessive sodium intake prompts aldosterone secretion, increasing fluid retention and blood pressure. Opt for a **low-sodium diet**, focusing on fresh vegetables, fruits, and whole grains, while minimizing processed foods and salt-heavy condiments.

2. **Maintain Optimal Potassium Levels:** Potassium has a counterbalancing effect on aldosterone and helps regulate blood pressure. Incorporate potassium-rich foods, such as **bananas, avocados, spinach**, and **sweet potatoes**, into your diet to support aldosterone balance and cardiovascular health.

3. **Hydrate Properly:** Dehydration triggers aldosterone release to conserve water and sodium. Ensuring adequate hydration is vital to prevent unnecessary aldosterone secretion. Drink enough water throughout the day, especially during periods of physical activity or hot weather.

4. **Exercise Regularly:** Physical activity not only supports heart and kidney health but also helps regulate aldosterone secretion. Regular **aerobic exercise** such as walking, running, swimming, or cycling helps manage blood pressure, improves fluid balance, and reduces stress, which in turn supports optimal aldosterone regulation.

5. **Stress Management:** Chronic stress can increase cortisol levels, which in turn can elevate aldosterone levels. Incorporating stress-reducing practices like **meditation**, **deep-breathing exercises**, and **mindfulness** into your daily routine can help keep aldosterone levels in check and support overall well-being.

6. **Genetic Testing and Personalized Care:** If you have a family history of aldosterone-related diseases, consider consulting with a healthcare provider about **genetic testing**. Identifying genetic mutations that affect aldosterone synthesis or receptor sensitivity can help tailor treatments and predict responses to medication.

7. **Consult a Healthcare Provider About Medication:** If you have been diagnosed with a condition involving aldosterone imbalances, such as **hypertension** or **heart failure**, working closely with your healthcare provider to determine the most appropriate pharmacological treatments is crucial. Be open to newer therapies that may offer fewer side effects and more effective outcomes.

Looking Toward the Future

As research into aldosterone continues to evolve, we are on the cusp of a new era in the treatment of related diseases. Advanced therapies, including **gene therapy**, **microRNA therapies**, and **novel receptor-targeting drugs**, offer promising pathways to more effective and personalized treatment options. The potential for **precision medicine**, which tailors treatment to the individual based on their genetic and environmental factors, will revolutionize the way we approach aldosterone imbalances and improve patient outcomes.

The future of aldosterone management holds exciting possibilities, and by continuing to explore and master this powerful hormone, we can unlock new opportunities for better health and longevity.

Final Thoughts: Maintaining Hormonal Balance for Longevity and Vitality

Mastering aldosterone is not just about managing disease; it is about optimizing **health** and **well-being**. By taking proactive steps to regulate aldosterone through diet, lifestyle, medication, and emerging therapies, we can significantly improve our health and quality of life.

Hormonal balance is key to maintaining a vibrant, healthy body, and aldosterone plays a crucial role in this process. By understanding its functions and its impact on our health, we can ensure that aldosterone works for us, not against us, paving the way for a long and healthy life.

Ultimately, the mastery of aldosterone is a journey—one that requires ongoing awareness, balanced choices, and personalized care. With the right approach, we can harness the power of aldosterone regulation to live life to its fullest, with vitality, resilience, and optimal health.

Chapter 25: Key Takeaways and Actionable Strategies

Throughout this book, we have explored the critical role of aldosterone in maintaining **fluid balance**, **blood pressure regulation**, and overall **hormonal health**. From its production and regulation to its impact on various organs, aldosterone serves as a key player in the body's intricate network of processes that keep us healthy. This final chapter will consolidate the essential takeaways and provide actionable strategies for mastering aldosterone, ensuring that it supports your health and wellness journey.

Key Takeaways:

1. **Aldosterone's Role in Fluid and Electrolyte Balance:** Aldosterone is crucial in regulating the balance of sodium, potassium, and water within the body. It promotes the retention of sodium in the kidneys, leading to increased fluid retention, which in turn raises blood volume and blood pressure. Proper regulation of aldosterone is essential to maintaining homeostasis and preventing both dehydration and excessive fluid accumulation.

2. **Blood Pressure Regulation and Hypertension:** Aldosterone's impact on blood pressure is profound. By promoting sodium retention, it can directly elevate blood pressure, contributing to **hypertension**. Conditions such as **primary aldosteronism** (Conn's syndrome) and **secondary hyperaldosteronism** are linked to excessive aldosterone production, increasing the risk of cardiovascular events, kidney damage, and strokes. Controlling aldosterone levels is crucial for managing these conditions.

3. **Aldosterone and the Heart:** Aldosterone plays a significant role in **cardiac remodeling** and heart failure. Elevated aldosterone levels contribute to increased fluid volume, which exacerbates the workload on the heart. **Aldosterone antagonists** like spironolactone and eplerenone have become essential therapies in treating heart failure, improving outcomes for many patients.

4. **Renal Function and Kidney Health:** In the kidneys, aldosterone regulates sodium and potassium balance. High aldosterone levels can lead to **kidney dysfunction** over time, especially in the presence of **chronic kidney disease** (CKD). On the other hand, aldosterone deficiency, as seen in **Addison's disease**, can result in dangerous electrolyte imbalances, highlighting the importance of careful aldosterone regulation in kidney health.

5. **Impact on Neurovascular Health:** Aldosterone also influences the **brain** and **neurovascular health**. Elevated aldosterone can increase the risk of **stroke** and contribute to cognitive decline by affecting the **blood-brain barrier**. As such, maintaining balanced aldosterone levels is crucial for both cardiovascular and cognitive health.

6. **The Interplay with Other Hormones:** The relationship between aldosterone and hormones like **cortisol** and **angiotensin II** is complex. Stress, chronic inflammation, and hormonal imbalances can all influence aldosterone secretion, leading to a cascade of effects that may exacerbate existing conditions like hypertension and kidney disease. Understanding these hormonal interactions is key to managing aldosterone levels effectively.

7. **Personalized Approaches to Treatment:** A growing area of research in aldosterone management involves **genetic testing** and **personalized medicine**. Genetic predispositions may affect how individuals respond to aldosterone-targeting drugs, making personalized care critical for effective treatment. Furthermore, advances in **aldosterone synthase inhibitors** and **microRNA therapies** could offer targeted solutions in the near future.

Actionable Strategies for Mastering Aldosterone:

1. **Monitor Sodium and Potassium Intake:** To keep aldosterone in check, maintaining a **balanced diet** is essential. High sodium intake triggers aldosterone secretion, while an adequate amount of **potassium** helps balance aldosterone's effects. Limit processed foods, and opt for fresh fruits, vegetables, and whole grains to support healthy aldosterone levels.

2. **Ensure Proper Hydration:** Dehydration can stimulate aldosterone production as the body attempts to conserve water. Ensure you are drinking enough water daily, especially if you engage in physical activity or live in a hot climate. Staying hydrated supports the body's natural ability to regulate aldosterone and other vital hormones.

3. **Exercise Regularly:** Regular exercise helps **reduce stress**, regulate aldosterone levels, and support cardiovascular health. **Aerobic exercises** such as walking, jogging, or swimming help promote healthy blood pressure levels and fluid balance. Exercise also improves **kidney function**, supporting aldosterone's role in renal health.

4. **Manage Stress Effectively:** Chronic stress increases **cortisol** and can lead to **elevated aldosterone**. Incorporating stress-reducing practices such as **meditation, yoga**, or **deep breathing** into your daily routine can help balance aldosterone and cortisol levels. Mindfulness techniques not only lower stress but also promote overall mental and physical well-being.

5. **Optimize Sleep Patterns:** Sleep is a crucial aspect of regulating hormonal balance. Lack of sleep can lead to increased aldosterone production and contribute to elevated blood pressure. Aim for **7-9 hours of quality sleep** per night to allow your body to recover and regulate hormones effectively.

6. **Consider Aldosterone Antagonists:** If you are diagnosed with **primary aldosteronism**, **hypertension**, or **heart failure**, discuss with your healthcare provider the use of **aldosterone antagonists** like **spironolactone** or **eplerenone**. These medications can help block the effects of aldosterone, reducing fluid retention and improving blood pressure control.

7. **Genetic Testing for Personalized Medicine:** If you have a family history of aldosterone-related conditions or are struggling to manage hypertension or kidney disease, consider genetic testing. Personalized care based on your genetic makeup can lead to more effective treatments and improve long-term health outcomes.

8. **Work with Healthcare Providers:** Regularly consult with your healthcare provider to monitor aldosterone levels, particularly if you have underlying conditions like **heart failure, hypertension**, or **chronic kidney disease**. By working closely with your doctor, you can tailor a treatment plan that includes **medications, lifestyle changes,** and **dietary adjustments** to optimize aldosterone balance.

The Future of Aldosterone Research and Treatment:

The future of aldosterone research is bright, with **targeted therapies** and **personalized treatments** paving the way for more precise management of aldosterone-related diseases. Advances in genetic testing, **gene therapy**, and **microRNA-based therapies** may provide groundbreaking treatments that specifically target aldosterone regulation.

Aldosterone's role in diseases like **hypertension**, **heart failure**, **kidney disease**, and even **cancer** will continue to be a key area of study, with new medications and interventions emerging as we learn more about its complex pathways.

As researchers continue to uncover the nuances of aldosterone's influence on the body, we can expect to see therapies that are more effective, with fewer side effects, offering hope for individuals who struggle with aldosterone-related health challenges.

Conclusion: Maintaining Hormonal Balance for Longevity and Vitality

Mastering aldosterone is not a singular task but an ongoing process that requires a holistic approach to health. From dietary choices and exercise to stress management and the latest pharmaceutical interventions, understanding aldosterone's role and how to regulate it can dramatically enhance your health and quality of life.

By applying the knowledge and strategies from this book, you can effectively manage aldosterone levels, preventing the complications associated with its imbalance, and unlocking the full potential of your body's hormonal system. Ultimately, mastering aldosterone is a key step toward achieving lasting health, vitality, and well-being.